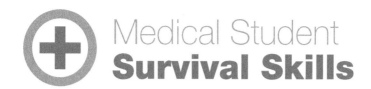

Medical Student
Survival Skills

Clinical
Examination

T0201441

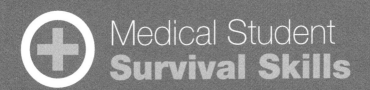

Medical Student
Survival Skills

Clinical
Examination

Philip Jevon RN BSc(Hons) PGCE
Academy Manager/Tutor
Walsall Teaching Academy, Manor Hospital, Walsall, UK

Elliot Epstein FRCP
Consultant Physician, Senior Academy Tutor
Walsall Healthcare NHS Trust, Manor Hospital, Walsall, UK

Sarah Mensforth FRCP
SpR in GU Medicine (West Midlands)
Walsall Healthcare NHS Trust, Manor Hospital, Walsall, UK

Caroline MacMahon FRCOG
SpR in Obstetrics & Gynaecology (West Midlands)
Walsall Healthcare NHS Trust, Manor Hospital, Walsall, UK

Consulting Editors

Jonathan Pepper BMedSci BM BS FRCOG MD FAcadMEd
Consultant Obstetrics and Gynaecology, Head of Academy
Walsall Healthcare NHS Trust, Manor Hospital, Walsall, UK

Jamie Coleman MBChB MD MA(Med Ed) FRCP FBPhS
Professor in Clinical Pharmacology and Medical Education / MBChB Deputy Programme
    Director
School of Medicine, University of Birmingham, Birmingham, UK

WILEY Blackwell

This edition first published 2020
© 2020 by John Wiley & Sons Ltd.

The right of Philip Jevon, Elliot Epstein, Sarah Mensforth, and Caroline MacMahon to be identified as the authors in this work has been asserted in accordance with law.

Registered Office(s)
John Wiley & Sons, Inc., 111 River Street, Hoboken, NJ 07030, USA
John Wiley & Sons Ltd, The Atrium, Southern Gate, Chichester, West Sussex, PO19 8SQ, UK

Editorial Office
9600 Garsington Road, Oxford, OX4 2DQ, UK

For details of our global editorial offices, customer services, and more information about Wiley products visit us at www.wiley.com.

Wiley also publishes its books in a variety of electronic formats and by print-on-demand. Some content that appears in standard print versions of this book may not be available in other formats.

Library of Congress Cataloging-in-Publication Data
Names: Jevon, Philip, author. | Epstein, Elliot (Consultant physician), author. |
  Mensforth, Sarah, author. | MacMahon, Caroline, author.
Title: Medical student survival skills. Clinical examination / Philip Jevon, Elliot Epstein, Sarah Mensforth,
  Caroline MacMahon.
Other titles: Clinical examination
Description: Hoboken, NJ : Wiley-Blackwell, 2020. | Includes index. | Identifiers: LCCN 2018060339 (print) |
  LCCN 2018061661 (ebook) | ISBN 9781118842041 (Adobe PDF) | ISBN 9781118842034 (ePub) |
  ISBN 9781118842010 (pbk.)
Subjects: | MESH: Physical Examination | Handbook
Classification: LCC RC78.7.D53 (ebook) | LCC RC78.7.D53 (print) | NLM WB 39 | DDC 616.07/54–dc23
LC record available at https://lccn.loc.gov/2018060339

Cover Design: Wiley
Cover Image: © WonderfulPixel/Shutterstock

Set in 9.25/12.5pt Helvetica Neue by SPi Global, Pondicherry, India

Printed in Great Britain by TJ International Ltd, Padstow, Cornwall

10 9 8 7 6 5 4 3 2 1

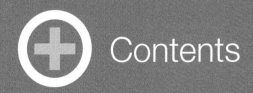 Contents

Acknowledgements

The authors are grateful to Steve Webb and Ishrat Ahmed for their help with the images and to Steve Webb, Anne DeBray, and Samrik Sandhu for their help with the website videos.

About the companion website

Don't forget to visit the companion website for this book:

www.wiley.com/go/jevon/medicalstudent

There you will find valuable material designed to enhance your learning, including:

- Videos
- Checklists

Scan this QR code to visit the companion website.

Examination of the cardiovascular system

1

NB Systematic approach: inspection, palpation, percussion, and auscultation.

Preparation

- *Cross infection*: wash and dry hands, bare below the elbow
- *Introductions*: yourself and the task; confirm patient's name and age
- *Consent*: to the procedure
- *Pain*: is the patient in pain
- *Privacy*: ensure privacy, e.g. curtains drawn around bed
- *Position*: ideally on the bed at 45° – if this is not possible, report that back to the observer
- *Exposure*: from the waist up, may not be appropriate to expose from the start of the exam for female patients

The peripheries

Inspection

- *Environment*: fluid restriction, glyceryl trinitrate (GTN) spray, oxygen, infusions, cardiac monitor
- *Patient*: breathlessness, distress, position, orthopnoea, pallor

NB Before you take their hand, double check again about pain.

Medical Student Survival Skills: Clinical Examination, First Edition. Philip Jevon, Elliot Epstein, Sarah Mensforth, and Caroline MacMahon.
© 2020 John Wiley & Sons Ltd. Published 2020 by John Wiley & Sons Ltd.
Companion website: www.wiley.com/go/jevon/medicalstudent

- *Hands*
  - Observe colour (pallor or peripheral cyanosis)
  - Feel for temperature
  - Measure capillary refill time (CRT) (Box 1.1): normal CRT <2 seconds
  - Look for tendon xanthomata (Figure 1.1), tar staining, clubbing, splinter haemorrhages (Figure 1.2), Janeway lesions, and Osler's nodes

Box 1.1 Measuring CRT

- Raise extremity (e.g. finger) slightly above the level of the heart
- Blanche the skin for 5 seconds and then release
- Note the CRT (normal is <2 seconds; prolonged CRT >2 seconds may be caused by circulatory shock, pyrexia, or a cool ambient temperature

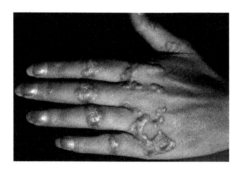

Figure 1.1 Tendon xanthomata – usually indicates hypercholesterolemia.

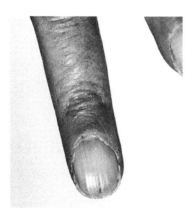

Figure 1.2 Splinter haemorrhages – may be seen in infective endocarditis.

OSCE Key Learning Points

✔ Stigmata of infective endocarditis include splinter haemorrhages, Janeway lesions/Osler's nodes, and clubbing

OSCE Key Learning Points

✔ Cardiac causes of clubbing include endocarditis and congenital heart disease

- *Face*
  - Look for malar flush (suggestive of mitral stenosis), central cyanosis (hypoxaemia), xanthelasma (hypercholesterolaemia) (Figure 1.3), corneal arcus (hypercholesterolaemia) (Figure 1.4), and pallor of the mucous membranes (anaemia)
- *Neck*
  - Observe the jugular venous pressure (JVP): position, waveform, and carotid pulsation
  - Measure the JVP (Figures 1.5a and b). The patient's position can affect JVP (Figure 1.5c)

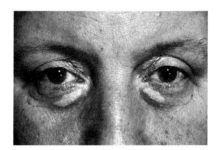

Figure 1.3 Xanthelasma – usually indicates hypercholesterolaemia.

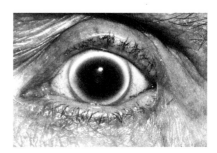

Figure 1.4 Corneal arcus – usually indicates hypercholesterolaemia.

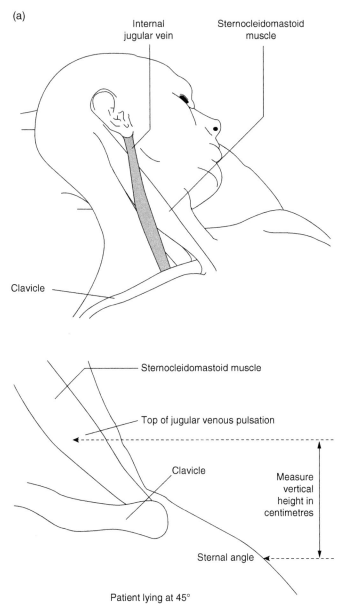

Figure 1.5 (a) Measurement of JVP: anatomy of the jugular veins and measuring the height of JVP. (b) Measurement of JVP. (c) The patient's position can affect JVP. Source: (a & c) Jevon, P. (2009). Clinical Examination Skills. Oxford: Wiley Blackwell. Reproduced with permission of Wiley.

(b)

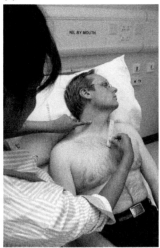

(c)

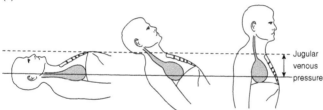

Figure 1.5 (Continued)

⚠ **Common misinterpretations and pitfalls**

The patient's position can significantly affect JVP (Figure 1.5c).

OSCE Key Learning Points ⊕

Cardiovascular causes of a raised JVP include

✔ Right-sided or congestive cardiac failure

✔ Cardiac tamponade

✔ Obstruction of superior vena cava, e.g. tumour

✔ Pulmonary embolism

✔ IV fluid overload

OSCE Key Learning Points

Distinguishing between a carotid pulse and JVP

✔ JVP moves down with inspiration, and rises with pressure on the right abdomen (liver: hepatojugular reflux – explain the procedure first!) and is impalpable

Palpation

- Pulses: palpate for 30 seconds
  - Palpate radial pulse or brachial pulse
  - Determine rate (bradycardia <60 beats per minute [bpm], tachycardia >100 bpm)
  - Assess rhythm (regular or irregular); if irregular, any pattern to irregularity or irregularly irregular
  - Assess pulse character at the carotid
  - Compare R + L for radioradial delay
  - Compare radial and femoral for radiofemoral delay
  - Assess for collapsing radial pulse (Box 1.2) – explain the procedure first!
- Request blood pressure (BP)

OSCE Key Learning Points

Four common causes of bradycardia

✔ Medications, e.g. beta-adrenoceptor blockers
✔ Ischaemic heart disease
✔ Hypothermia
✔ Normal finding, e.g. athletes

OSCE Key Learning Points

Four common causes of tachycardia

✔ Medications, e.g. salbutamol
✔ Ischaemic heart disease
✔ Circulatory shock
✔ Exercise/anxiety

> **Box 1.2 Assessing for a collapsing pulse (a marker of aortic regurgitation)**
>
> - Explain to the patient they will need to lift their arm swiftly upwards – check about shoulder pain and movement limitations first
> - Stand to the side of the patient
> - Locate the radial pulse with your fingertips. Then adjust so the flat of your palm around the first metacarpophangeal (MCP) joint is flush against the pulse area
> - Swiftly elevate and straighten the arm: a collapsing pulse is felt against your hand – normally the pulse will not be palpable in this position

 NB Do not forget to ask for the BP – it can give you clues if you hear a murmur later!

The precordium

Inspection

- Look for scars (coronary artery bypass graft (CABG), drains, implantable cardiac devices (ICDs), chest wall deformities, visible heaves or pulsations
- If a median sternotomy scar is present, check the calves for vein graft harvest (their presence suggests that the sternotomy scar relates to CABG)

Palpation

- Palpate the apex beat using the finger tips. This is normally located in 5th intercostal space (ICS), mid-clavicular line. Ensure you demonstrate finding the location by counting the rib spaces. Note the rhythm and character of the apex beat (Box 1.3). If the apex beat is displaced, check the trachea. If also displaced this indicates mediastinal shift
- Check for heaves and thrills using the flat of your hand

> **Box 1.3 Character of the apex beat**
>
> *Normal*: short and sharp
> *Heaving*: sustained and forceful due to an obstruction to the flow of blood out of the heart, e.g. aortic stenosis
> *Thrusting*: volume overload
> *Tapping*: mitral stenosis
> *Diffuse*: left ventricular failure and cardiomypathy

OSCE Key Learning Points

Causes of an impalpable apex include
- ✔ High body mass index (BMI)
- ✔ Emphysema
- ✔ Pericardial effusion
- ✔ Dextrocardia

Auscultation (Figure 1.6)

- At the apex – left 5th ICS, mid-clavicular line normally
- At the mitral area (M) – left 5th ICS, mid-clavicular line
- At the tricuspid area (T) – left 4th ICS, lateral to the sternum
- At the pulmonary area (P) – left 2nd ICS, lateral to the sternum
- At the aortic area (A) – right 2nd ICS, lateral to the sternum
  Auscultate for S1 and S2 in each area:
    - Check that S1 matches with the carotid pulse in the neck (Figure 1.7). This skill will take practice, but is important
    - Once you have identified S1 and S2, listen between the sounds for murmurs

Perform the manoeuvres for each murmur as routine, whilst you progress through the four areas, or afterwards. In the mitral area:
- Roll the patient into the left lateral to amplify a mitral murmur
- Listen with the bell (mitral stenosis [MS])
- Listen in the axilla (radiation of mitral regurgitation [MR])

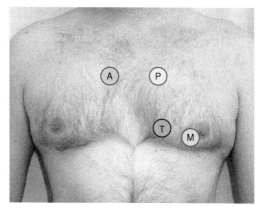

Figure 1.6 Auscultation of the precordium.

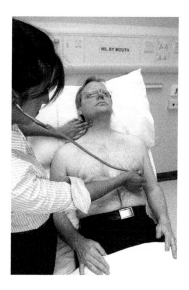

Figure 1.7 Checking that S1 matches with the carotid pulse in the neck.

For aortic murmurs:

- Listen to the carotid area of the neck for murmur radiation (of aortic stenosis [AS])
- Ask to sit forwards, place your stethoscope at the lower left sternal edge (LLSE) and then listen in end-expiration (radiation of aortic regurgitation [AR])

For any murmur (Table 1.1):

- Listen in inspiration and expiration:
  - Left-sided murmurs (aortic and mitral) become louder in expiration
  - Right-sided murmurs (pulmonary and tricuspid) become louder in inspiration

Table 1.1 Characteristics of Common Murmurs

	Aortic stenosis	Aortic regurgitation	Mitral stenosis	Mitral regurgitation
Systolic/diastolic?	Ejection systolic	Early diastolic	Mid diastolic	Pan systolic
Loudest at ...?	R 2nd ICS	LLSE	L 5th ICS	L 5th ICS
Manoeuvre	Listen at carotid	Listen at LLSE leaning forward in end expiration	Listen with the bell	Roll to left lateral
Radiation?	Carotids	LLSE	–	Axilla
Effect on apex?	Heaving, Undisplaced	Displaced, Hyperdynamic	Tapping	Hyperdynamic
Effect on pulse?	Slow rising	Collapsing	None	None
Effect on BP?	Narrowed	Widened	None	None

Other sounds:

- S3 – a low pitched sound heard just after S2. It can be normal in young fit people or pregnancy, or a sign of left ventricular function impairment and dilation
- S4 – a low pitched heart sound just before S1. This indicates forceful atrial contraction against stiff ventricles, and is always abnormal
- Pericardial friction rub – often described as a creaking sound similar to walking on firm snow; due to pericarditis. Ask the patient to hold their breath to make this more audible

Ken – – – tuck – y S1 – – – S2 – S3 T – enne – – – ssee S4 – S1 – – – S2	The rhythm of the words 'Kentucky' and 'Tennessee' are often used to remember the added sounds' timing relative to S1 and S2

Auscultation continued

- Whilst they lean forward (as you check for AR):
  - Auscultate the lung bases for signs of pulmonary oedema
  - Inspect and palpate for sacral oedema

To complete the examination

- Inspect the legs for oedema, scars, ulcers and trophic changes
- Request blood pressure
- Offer to check radioradial and radiofemoral delay (if not done earlier)
- Examine the other peripheral pulses
- Perform a peripheral vascular examination – if appropriate
- Thank the patient
- Cover the patient up and ensure they are comfortable
- Request appropriate investigations, e.g. oxygen saturations and electro-cardiogram (ECG)

OSCE Key Learning Points

Cardiovascular system: example presentation

✔ On examination round the bed I note that there is GTN spray at the bedside. This elderly gentleman appears comfortable sitting upright.

✔ On examination of the peripheries there are no signs of infective endocarditis or heart failure, I do note corneal arcus of the eye. The pulse has a normal volume and regular rhythm at a rate of 78 bpm. The blood pressure is 146/86 mmHg.

✔ On examination of the precordium, there were no scars, heaves nor thrills. I could hear heart sounds 1 and 2, with an added murmur. This was systolic and loudest in the aortic area. Its character was ejection systolic, and I conclude that this could be aortic stenosis.

✔ To complete the examination I would examine the peripheral pulses and inspect the legs, which I did not manage to complete in the time allowed.

Examination of the respiratory system

2

NB Systematic approach: inspection, palpation, percussion, and auscultation.

Preparation

- *Cross infection*: wash and dry hands, bare below the elbow
- *Introductions*: yourself and the task; confirm patient's name and age
- *Consent*: to the procedure
- *Pain*: is the patient in pain
- *Privacy*: ensure privacy, e.g. curtains drawn around bed
- *Position*: ideally on the bed at 45° – if this is not possible, report that back to the observer
- *Exposure*: from the waist up, may not be appropriate to expose from the start of the exam for female patients

The peripheries

Inspection

- *Environment*: inhalers, steroid card, nebuliser, oxygen (note delivery devices and flow rate), or sputum pot
- *Patient*: breathlessness, cachexia, pursed lip breathing, markers of respiratory distress such as intercostal recession, a splinting/bracing sitting position

NB Before you take their hand, double check again about pain.

Medical Student Survival Skills: Clinical Examination, First Edition. Philip Jevon, Elliot Epstein, Sarah Mensforth, and Caroline MacMahon.
© 2020 John Wiley & Sons Ltd. Published 2020 by John Wiley & Sons Ltd.
Companion website: www.wiley.com/go/jevon/medicalstudent

- *Hands*
  - Observe colour (peripheral cyanosis), tar staining, clubbing (Figure 2.1), palmar erythema, bruising, and dilated veins
  - Observe for fine tremor (can be induced by beta-2 agonist therapy)
  - Assess for CO_2 retention flap for at least 15 seconds (Figure 2.2)
  - Feel for temperature, radial pulse (30 seconds), and capillary refill time (CRT) (see Box 1.1) – explain the procedure first

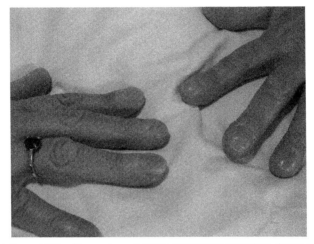

Figure 2.1 Finger clubbing. Source: Jevon, P. (2009). Clinical Examination Skills. Oxford: Wiley Blackwell. Reproduced with permission of Wiley.

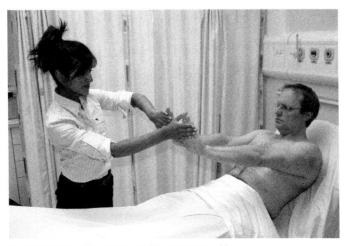

Figure 2.2 Assessing for CO_2 retention flap (at least 15 seconds).

NB Whilst palpating the radial pulse, this is a good time to assess respiratory rate – if you *tell* the patient you are counting their breathing rate they will alter the rate subconsciously!

OSCE Key Learning Points

✔ Stigmata of CO_2 retention include tremor, venodilation (dorsum of hands, chemosis of eyes) and, in extreme cases, convulsions

OSCE Key Learning Points

Respiratory causes of clubbing include

✔ Suppurative lung disease (bronchiectasis, empyema, cystic fibrosis)

✔ Lung cancer including mesothelioma

✔ Pulmonary fibrosis

- *Face*
  - Look for plethora, moon face, central cyanosis, chemosis, corneal arcus, and pallor of the mucous membranes (indicating anaemia)
- *Neck*
  - Look for the jugular venous pressure (JVP) position and waveform (see Figure 1.5)
  - Palpate the trachea
    - If this is *not* central, palpate the apex. If both are displaced, this indicates mediastinal displacement
    - Measure the distance between the sternal notch and the cricoid cartilage: three to four finger breadths in expiration is normal; it is chronically reduced in patients with emphysematous and hyperexpanded lungs
  - Palpate for cervical lymph nodes – this can also be done at the end of the exam

The chest

Inspection

- Look for scars (thoracotomy, drain, and tracheostomy scars), chest wall deformities, kyphosis, scoliosis, barrel chest, pectus excavatum, and pectus carinatum, drains, dressings
- If you have not yet counted respiratory rate, do so now

OSCE Key Learning Points

✔ You may choose to perform all skills (palpation, percussion, and auscultation) on the anterior chest then move to the posterior chest

✔ You may prefer to perform each skill on the anterior then move to the posterior aspect of the chest

Palpation

- Assess lung expansion (Figure 2.3) in two places, anteriorly and posteriorly. Note extent and symmetry of expansion
- Anterior:
  - Place the palms of the hands over the upper part of the anterior chest wall and observe for anterior and upward expansion
  - Loosely grasp the chest with fingertips in the lower rib spaces on either side of the chest. Bring the thumbs to the centre and use their movement as a marker of lateral expansion. The thumbs should not rest on the chest
- Posterior – test for lateral expansion as above

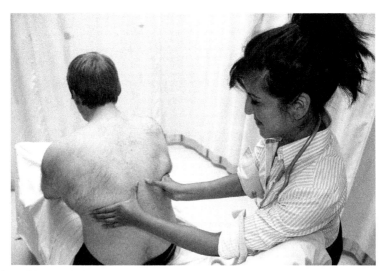

Figure 2.3 Assessing lung expansion.

OSCE Key Learning Points

✔ For percussion and auscultation we suggest you examine 2–3 areas anteriorly, 1–2 in the axilla and 3–4 posteriorly left and right (Figure 2.4)

(a)

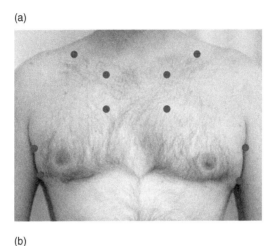

(b)

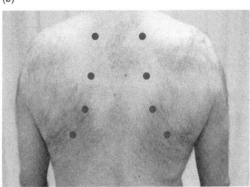

Figure 2.4 (a and b) Suggested areas for percussion and auscultation.

Percussion

- Examine in each area top to bottom, right to left, comparing the 'note'.
- Place the non-dominant hand on the chest wall with the middle finger pressed against the area to be percussed. Gently strike the middle phalanx of that finger with the middle fingertip of the other hand (Figure 2.5)

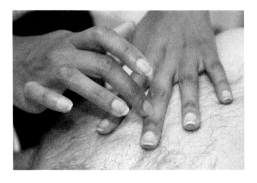

Figure 2.5 Chest percussion technique.

OSCE Key Learning Points

✔ Causes of dullness to percussion include consolidation, collapse, and effusion (stony dull)

✔ Causes of hyper-resonance to percussion include pneumothorax and emphysema

Auscultation

● Examine in each area top to bottom, right to left, comparing the breath sounds, and listening for bronchial breathing and added sounds, such as crackles, wheeze, and rubs

● Ensure you hear inspiratory and expiratory phases of breathing

OSCE Key Learning Points

✔ Causes of wheeze include chronic obstructive pulmonary disease, asthma, and heart failure

✔ Causes of crackles include pneumonia (coarse crackles), pulmonary oedema, and pulmonary fibrosis (fine crackles)

✔ Causes of bronchial breathing include consolidation and collapse

To complete the examination

● If you have not counted the respiratory rate, do this now

● Check the calves for evidence of deep vein thrombosis

● Offer to check cervical lymph nodes

- Offer to perform peak expiratory flow rate if wheeze is present
- Thank the patient
- Cover the patient up and ensure they are comfortable
- Request oxygen saturations
- Request electrocardiogram (ECG) or chest X-ray

 Common misinterpretations and pitfalls

Going too slow and not getting to the end of the examination, so could start on the back.

OSCE Key Learning Points

Respiratory system: example presentation

✔ I examined this elderly gentleman's respiratory system. At the bedside, I noted that there is a nebuliser box, and that the patient is receiving oxygen therapy at $2 l min^{-1}$. From the end of the bed, I can see that this gentleman is tachypnoeic, with a rate of 24 breaths per minute. On examination of the peripheries, he has signs of peripheral cyanosis. There is no flap to indicate CO_2 retention. There are no other signs of respiratory disease.

✔ On examination of the chest, there are no obvious scars or drains. Expansion was reduced in the right lower zone on the posterior aspect of the chest. At this area there is dullness to percussion, stony dull, and there are reduced breath sounds. Vocal resonance was similarly reduced in the right lower zone on the posterior aspect. This gentleman may have a right-sided pleural effusion.

✔ To complete the examination I would assess oxygen saturations and examine the cervical lymph nodes.

3 Examination of the gastrointestinal system

 NB Systematic approach: inspection, palpation, percussion, and auscultation.

Preparation

- *Cross infection*: wash and dry hands, bare below the elbow
- *Introductions*: yourself and the task; confirm patient's name and age
- *Consent*: to the procedure
- *Pain*: is the patient in pain
- *Privacy*: ensure privacy, e.g. curtains drawn around bed
- *Position*: initially on the bed at 45° – if this is not possible, report that back to the observer
- *Exposure*: ideally from nipples to knees, state this to the examiner. In the exam, you may preserve the dignity of the patient by limiting your exposure from the xiphisternum to the pubic symphysis

The peripheries

End of bed inspection
- *Environment*: fluid restriction, intravenous infusion, vomit bowl, food/supplements
- *Patient*:
  - Pain: distress
  - Position: are they lying still with legs pulled up, which may suggest peritonitis, or moving around unable to get comfortable, which can indicate renal colic

Medical Student Survival Skills: Clinical Examination, First Edition. Philip Jevon, Elliot Epstein, Sarah Mensforth, and Caroline MacMahon.
© 2020 John Wiley & Sons Ltd. Published 2020 by John Wiley & Sons Ltd.
Companion website: www.wiley.com/go/jevon/medicalstudent

- Nutritional state: obesity/cachexia
- Colour, e.g. jaundice, pallor

OSCE Key Learning Points

✔ Your end of bed assessment of the patient is essential both in exams and in clinical practice, so ensure you are thorough and methodical. It is also the first impression you give to the examiner!

Hands

- Temperature: with the back of your hands
- Capillary refill time
- Nails: koilonychia (Figure 3.1), leuconychia, and clubbing
- Palms: palmar erythema (Figure 3.2) and Dupytren's contracture
- Hepatic asterixis (liver flap): ask the patient to extend their arms straight in front of them and extend their wrists upwards (see Figure 2.2). Hold for 15 seconds, with gentle pressure on the fingers applying dorsiflexion to the wrist. A liver flap produces a slow, twitching flexion of the fingers and wrist, and is characteristic of hepatic encephalopathy

⚠ Common misinterpretations and pitfalls

Assessing for liver flap for < 15 seconds is not sufficient and may result in a liver flap not being observed.

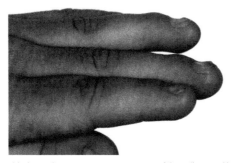

Figure 3.1 Koilonychia (spooning or concave appearance of the nail caused by severe iron deficiency).

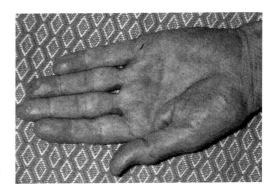

Figure 3.2 Palmar erythema (can be associated with liver failure).

OSCE Key Learning Points

Gastrointestinal causes of clubbing include

✔ Hepatic cirrhosis

✔ Coeliac disease

✔ Inflammatory bowel disease (Crohn's and ulcerative colitis)

Arms

- Pulse: rate and rhythm.
- Bruising (many clotting factors are synthesised in the liver, thus liver failure may cause prolonged clotting time)
- Excoriations
- Needle marks (IV drug use: risk factor for hepatitis B and C)
- Tattoos (risk factor for hepatitis B and C)
- Blood pressure (many pathologies causing abdominal pain may lead to shock)

OSCE Key Learning Points

✔ Stigmata of chronic liver disease include: jaundice, bruising, asterixis, spider naevi, gynaecomastia, ascites, caput medusae, splenomegaly, pedal oedema, and encephalopathy

Face

- *Eyes*: jaundice, xanthelasma, corneal arcus, and conjunctival pallor
- *Mouth*: angular stomatitis and glossitis (B_{12}/folate deficiency), apthous ulcers, hydration status, telangiectasia (hereditary haemorrhagic telangiectasia), perioral pigmentation (Peutz–Jeghers syndrome)

Neck

- Jugular venous pressure
- Virchow's node (left supraclavicular – associated with gastric cancer) (Figure 3.3)

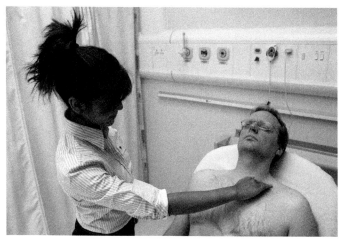

Figure 3.3 Palpating Virchow's node (Troisier's sign).

OSCE Key Learning Points

Causes of jaundice include

✔ Pre-hepatic: haemolytic anaemia

✔ Hepatocellular: viral hepatitis, alcoholic liver disease, steatohepatitis, autoimmune hepatitis, toxins (e.g. paracetamol)

✔ Post-hepatic (i.e. obstructive): choledocholithiasis, malignancy (head of pancreas or cholangiocarcinoma), primary biliary cholangitis

Chest

- Gynaecomastia
- Spider naevi (Figure 3.4)

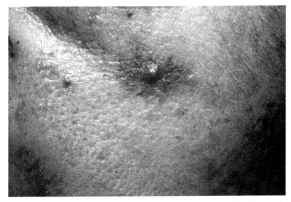

Figure 3.4 Spider naevi (can be normal finding; five or more is considered a sign of chronic liver disease).

The abdomen

OSCE Key Learning Points

When examining the abdomen
- ✔ Ask first if they are comfortable to lie flat
- ✔ Lie the patient flat
- ✔ Position yourself level with the patient, either by crouching down or raising the bed
- ✔ Observe their face for pain throughout your palpation

Inspection

Begin by asking the patient to cough, which may unmask any hernias. Lifting their head may reveal divarification of the rectus. Then go on to inspect for the following:
- Distension
- Scars: location, estimate their age, suggest what surgery they may indicate (Figure 3.5)
- Distended veins
- Bruising (Cullen's and Grey Turner's signs)
- Drains: position, health of insertion site, bag contents (colour, volume)
- Stomas

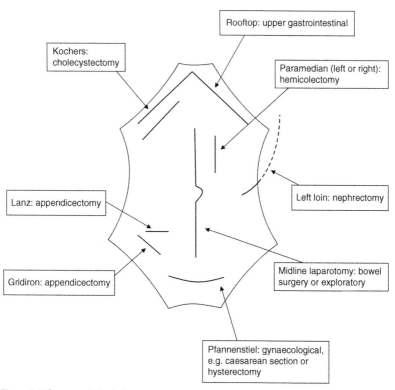

Figure 3.5 Common abdominal scars.

 NB Cullen's and Grey Turner's signs: acute pancreatitis can cause haemorrhage into the retroperitoneal space. Blood-stained fluid may then track to the skin around the umbilicus (Cullen's sign) or at the flanks (Grey Turner's sign). These are both signs of severe disease.

 Common misinterpretations and pitfalls

Do not forget to inspect closely for small scars of a previous laparoscopy, which may be difficult to see. These will be around a centimetre in length and found inferior to the umbilicus, as well as in the outer quadrants.

OSCE Key Learning Points

Causes of abdominal distension: the five 'F's
- ✔ Fat
- ✔ Faeces
- ✔ Flatus
- ✔ Fluid
- ✔ Foetus

Palpation
- *Superficial*: gentle palpation in the nine quadrants, to assess pain and signs of peritonism (guarding and rebound tenderness) (Figure 3.6). Start away from any source of pain
- *Deep*: palpation in the nine quadrants examining for masses
- *Murphy's sign* (if relevant): a sign of cholecystitis. Pain on deep inspiration while palpating in the right upper quadrant (RUQ). It is only positive if absent on the left
- *Liver*: from right iliac fossa (RIF), moving towards the RUQ as the patient breathes in and out. Ensure your palpation corresponds to the patient's inspiration, when the liver moves inferiorly. If a liver edge is felt, describe it: e.g. smooth/irregular/tender
- *Spleen*: also start in RIF, moving towards the left upper quadrant (LUQ) with each inspiration

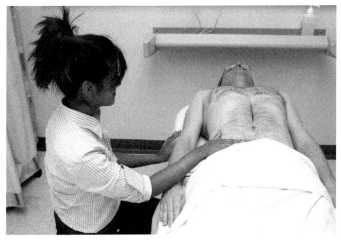

Figure 3.6 Palpation of the abdomen.

- *Kidneys*: ballot bilaterally, ensuring hand is sufficiently posterior (behind the patient's loin)
- *Abdominal aortic aneurysm (AAA)* (Figure 3.7): expansile and pulsatile mass. The bifurcation of the aorta into the common iliac vessels is at the level of the umbilicus, so ensure you palpate above this landmark. Presentation of an AAA is clinically variable, so it is essential to consider in all causes of acute abdominal pain
- *Abdominal masses:* Figure 3.8 details the location of common abdominal masses

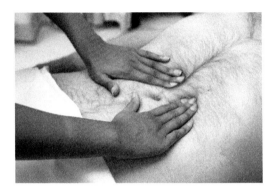

Figure 3.7 Palpation for an abdominal aortic aneurysm.

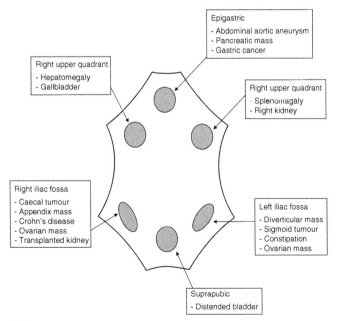

Epigastric
- Abdominal aortic aneurysm
- Pancreatic mass
- Gastric cancer

Right upper quadrant
- Hepatomegaly
- Gallbladder

Right upper quadrant
- Splenomagaly
- Right kidney

Right iliac fossa
- Caecal tumour
- Appendix mass
- Crohn's disease
- Ovarian mass
- Transplanted kidney

Left iliac fossa
- Diverticular mass
- Sigmoid tumour
- Constipation
- Ovarian mass

Suprapubic
- Distended bladder

Figure 3.8 Common abdominal masses.

OSCE Key Learning Points

Distinguishing the kidney from the spleen

✔ The kidney has no notch

✔ You can get above the kidney

✔ Kidneys are ballotable (will bounce against you upper hand when palpated from below)

NB Biliary disease:

- *Courvoisier's law*: 'in the presence of jaundice, a palpable gallbladder is unlikely to be due to gallstones', i.e. it is more likely to be caused by an obstructing malignancy. This is because cholecystitis leads to fibrosis of the gallbladder, therefore it usually distends less
- *Charcot's triad*: Fever, jaundice, and RUQ pain. Consistent with ascending cholangitis

Percussion

- Liver:
  - Lower border: from RIF to RUQ
  - Upper border: from right 5th intercostal space, mid-clavicular line (liver may be displaced inferiorly in lung hyperexpansion caused by respiratory disease)
- Spleen: in a line from RIF to LUQ
- If you find enlargement of either of these organs, describe the extension below the costal margin in centimetres
- Shifting dullness for ascites if the abdomen is distended

OSCE Key Learning Points

Examining for ascites by 'shifting dullness'

✔ With the patient lying flat, percuss in a straight line from the umbilicus towards the left flank, until a dull percussion note is detected

✔ Keeping a finger in the same spot, ask the patient to roll towards you

✔ Wait for 10 seconds and percuss again in that spot

✔ If the note is now resonant, the fluid has shifted, indicating the presence of ascites

Auscultation

- Bowel sounds: high tinkling bowel sounds are suggestive of obstruction. Reduced or absent bowel sounds may be observed in paralytic ileus or peritonitis
- Renal bruits: renal artery stenosis (an uncommonly detected sign)

Examination of a stoma

Preparation

- Gloves
- If practical it is best to remove the bag for a close inspection (always check the patient has another one available)
- Be familiar with the characteristics of stomas (Table 3.1)

Table 3.1 Characteristics of Stomas

	Ileostomy	Colostomy
Position (may vary)	RIF	Usually RUQ or left lower quadrant
Appearance	Spout	Flush with skin
Output	Liquid	Usually more formed

Inspection

- Site
- Colour of the bowel mucosa
- Health of the surrounding skin
- Bag contents: volume, colour, consistency
- Other scars on the abdomen which may suggest the underlying procedure. Laparotomy or laparoscopy scars or any round scars which might suggest previous stoma sites

Palpation

- Around stoma for hernias (ask patient to cough)

Other types of stoma

- *Loop ileostomy* (Figure 3.9) or *colostomy*: features are as above, but with afferent and efferent limbs, and therefore a double lumen. This is a 'defunctioning' stoma, with the intention to reconnect the bowel at a later date. The second lumen may be difficult to visualise
- *Mucous fistula*: the non-functioning end of the bowel. The same principle as a loop colostomy, but with the inactive side brought out at a different location. Allows passage of mucous and flatus, which may accumulate in

the distal segment of the bowel, and allows easy location of the end for later re-anastomosis

- *Urostomy:* these are uncommon, and usually performed due to a neurogenic bladder (e.g. spina bifida) or following cystectomy due to malignancy. They are similar in appearance to an ileostomy (and in fact are formed from an ileal conduit), but the contents of the bag will be urine

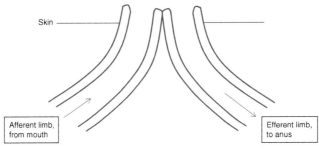

Skin

Afferent limb, from mouth

Efferent limb, to anus

Figure 3.9 Loop ileostomy.

OSCE Key Learning Points

Complications of stomas include

- ✔ Anatomical: retraction, stenosis, hernia, prolapse
- ✔ Vascular: haemorrhage, ischaemia, necrosis
- ✔ Dermatological: irritant dermatitis (ileostomy)
- ✔ Functional: high output, electrolyte abnormalities
- ✔ Psychological: psychosexual disturbance

Hernial orifices

Palpate the inguinal regions bilaterally and ask the patient to cough. If a mass is felt, describe it according to the generic structure in Chapter 4 describing examination of the groin. If you find a groin swelling which you suspect is a hernia, stand the patient up and examine it as follows.

Inspection
- Site
- Size
- Overlying skin: erythema may indicate strangulation
- Any scars: have they had a previous repair?

Palpation

- Tenderness
- Cough impulse
- Test for direct versus indirect

Auscultation

- Bowel sounds

OSCE Key Learning Points

Causes of a groin mass include

✔ Inguinal hernia

✔ Femoral hernia

✔ Undescended testis

✔ Femoral aneurysm

✔ Saphenous varix

✔ Lymph node

OSCE Key Learning Points

Complications of inguinal hernias include

✔ Incarceration: non-reducible

✔ Obstruction: mechanical blockage of bowel in the hernia

✔ Strangulation: ischaemia of tissue within the hernia, due to venous congestion

OSCE Key Learning Points

Complications of inguinal hernia repair include

✔ Immediate: haemorrhage, nerve damage (ilioinguinal)

✔ Short term: infection, urinary retention, scrotal haematoma

✔ Late: recurrence, ischaemic orchitis

To complete the examination

- Inspect legs for oedema and rashes
- Cervical and inguinal lymphadenopathy if indicated
- Ask for observations and fluid balance chart
- Offer to examine the hernial orifices and external genitalia
- Offer to perform a digital rectal examination if indicated
- Thank the patient
- Cover the patient up and ensure they are comfortable

OSCE Key Learning Points

Gastrointestinal system: example presentation

✔ I examined Mrs Jones, a 54-year-old lady who presented with abdominal distension. On end of bed inspection, she was alert and orientated and comfortable at rest, cachectic in appearance, and there was obvious jaundice.

✔ Around the bed I noted an empty vomit bowl and a urinary catheter containing 100 ml of clear urine. On examination of the peripheries, there was leukonychia, bruising, yellow sclera, and spider naevi, but no hepatic asterixis was observed. On inspection of the abdomen there was marked symmetrical distension.

✔ On palpation the abdomen was soft and non-tender, with a smooth, tender liver edge felt 4 cm below the costal margin, and confirmed on percussion. There was no splenomegaly. Shifting dullness was positive, indicating the presence of ascites.

✔ In summary, this lady displays signs consistent with chronic liver disease, but clinically there is no encephalopathy. I would like to examine her observations and fluid balance chart, and order baseline investigations starting with bloods tests, including full blood count, urea and electrolytes, liver function tests, C-reactive protein, and clotting.

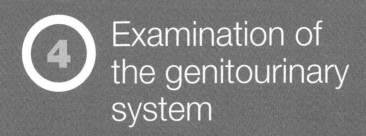

Examination of the genitourinary system

NB Systematic approach: inspection and palpation.

Preparation

- *Cross infection*: wash and dry hands, bare below the elbow
- *Introductions*: yourself and the task; confirm patient's name and age
- *Consent*: to the procedure; this is particularly important in any examination of the genitalia. Ensure you explain what your examination entails and what you are looking for
- *Pain*: is the patient in pain
- *Privacy*: ensure privacy, e.g. curtains drawn around bed
- *Chaperone*: this is essential for any genital examination, and you must document the name of your chaperone
- *Position*: patient standing, with student kneeling to their right (Figure 4.1). If this is not possible, report that back to the observer
- *Exposure*: ideally from waist down

NB A chaperone should be present.

Medical Student Survival Skills: Clinical Examination, First Edition. Philip Jevon, Elliot Epstein, Sarah Mensforth, and Caroline MacMahon.
© 2020 John Wiley & Sons Ltd. Published 2020 by John Wiley & Sons Ltd.
Companion website: www.wiley.com/go/jevon/medicalstudent

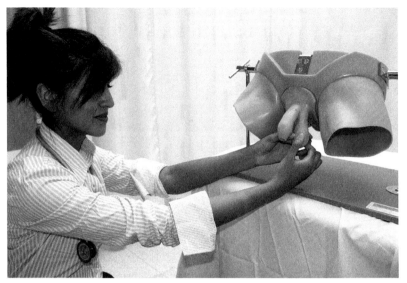

Figure 4.1 Position for examination of the groin.

End of bed inspection

- *Environment*: urinary bottle/bedpan, urinary catheter, IV fluids
- *Patient*:
  - Pain, distress. Do they look well?
  - Body mass index (BMI): any cachexia?

NB Even in a focused examination such as the groin, it is essential to consider the whole patient. You may detect cachexia in a patient with malignancy, or a patient with an obstructed inguinal hernia may be tachypnoeic and distressed with abdominal distension.

OSCE Key Learning Points

✔ Starting your examination with the patient standing will allow better detection of hernias and varicocoeles

OSCE Key Learning Points

Causes of acutely painful testicular swelling include

✔ Testicular torsion

✔ Epididymo-orchitis

✔ Acute haematocoele

 NB Remember that the testicles drain to the para-aortic lymph nodes, while the penis and scrotum drain to the inguinal nodes. The prostate drains to the internal iliac nodes.

The groin

Inspection

Begin by asking the patient to cough, which may unmask any hernias. Then go on to inspect for the following.

- *Scrotum*
  - Swelling: any asymmetry
  - Look for scars: location, estimate their age, suggest what surgery they may be from
  - Erythema
  - Rashes or ulcers
  - Lift the scrotum with the back of your hand to inspect the posterior aspect and the perineum
- *Penis*
  - Inspect the glans for ulcers, phimosis, erythema, and discharge, retracting the foreskin (do not forget to replace)
  - Confirm anatomical location of the urethral meatus (hypospadias causes opening to be located along the shaft of the penis)

Palpation

- *Testicles*: normal first. Stabilise between finger and thumb of non-dominant hand (Figure 4.2), while gently palpating the entire surface with the other hand
- *Epididymis:* on the posterior aspect of the testicle
- *Spermatic cord:* follow this superiorly as far as you can
- *Inguinal lymphadenopathy*

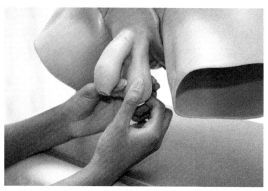

Figure 4.2 Palpation of the testes.

Examination of a lump

This general examination structure can be applied to any mass (Figure 4.3).

Inspection
Inspect the six 'S's, if not already covered:

- Site
- Size
- Shape
- Symmetry
- Skin
- Scars

Palpation

- Temperature: with the back of your hand
- Tenderness
- Surface: smooth or irregular
- Edge: diffuse or well circumscribed
- Consistency: hard, firm, or soft; rubbery
- Mobility: is it mobile or fixed to surrounding structures. If fixed, what to?
- Fluctuance: indicates fluid
- Pulsatility
- Reducibility
- Transilluminability
- Cough impulse: absence of this does not rule out hernia, as the hernia may lose cough impulse when incarcerated

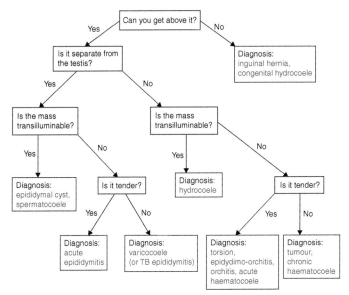

Figure 4.3 Examination of a testicular lump.

NB Fluctuance is a clinical sign indicating the presence of a fluid collection within the tissue, for example a hydrocele or an abscess. It can be assessed by placing the thumb and index finger of one hand on either side of the swelling. Pressing with the index finger of the opposite hand in the centre of the lump will displace your fingers laterally, indicating fluid.

Features of a testicular lump

- Can you get above it (Figure 4.3)
- Is there a cough impulse
- Are the testes palpable

Figure 4.4 shows a classification of the different kinds of testicular lumps.

To complete the examination

- Thank the patient
- Ensure the patient is covered up
- Order a mid-stream specimen of urine (MSU)

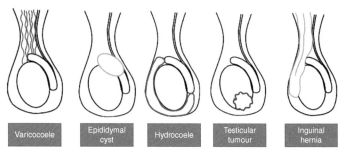

| Varicocoele | Epididymal cyst | Hydrocoele | Testicular tumour | Inguinal hernia |

Figure 4.4 Classification of testicular lumps.

- Inguinal lymphadenopathy if not done
- Offer to perform full abdominal examination
- Offer to perform a digital rectal examination
- Order ultrasound scan

OSCE Key Learning Points

Genitourinary system: example presentation

✔ Today I have performed a testicular examination of Mr Jones. On general inspection he was alert and orientated, and comfortable at rest. Body habitus showed increased BMI, but there were no obvious peripheral indicators of disease.

✔ On inspection of the scrotum there was asymmetry with a swelling of roughly 6 cm located in the right hemi-scrotum, however there was no erythema, skin changes or overlying scars.

✔ On palpation the swelling was smooth-surfaced, non-tender, soft in consistency, and with a well-circumscribed edge. It was mobile within the skin of the scrotum but fixed to the testicle, and was found to transilluminate. It was located at the superior aspect of the scrotum, and was separate from the testicle. It was possible to get above the lump and it did not demonstrate a cough impulse.

✔ There were no abnormalities noted in the penis and no inguinal lymphadenopathy. These findings would be consistent with an epididymal cyst.

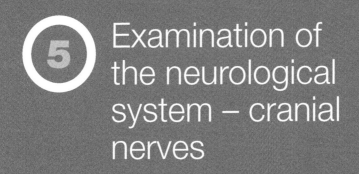

5 Examination of the neurological system – cranial nerves

OSCE Key Learning Points

✔ Remember to spend time inspecting from the end of the bed

Preparation

- *Cross infection*: wash and dry hands, bare below the elbow
- *Introductions*: yourself and the task; confirm patient's name and age
- *Consent*: to the procedure
- *Pain*: is the patient in pain
- *Privacy*: ensure privacy, e.g. curtains drawn around bed
- *Position*: sitting in a chair or on a bed
- *Exposure*: head and neck

Inspection

- *Environment*: wheelchair, crutches, orthopaedic shoes, hearing aids, spectacles.
- *Patient*: positioning, posture, facial features or asymmetry

 NB To achieve a slick, confident performance, practice giving the instructions to *patients* – your peers will know what to do even if your instructions are not clear, patients will need extremely clear instructions.

Medical Student Survival Skills: Clinical Examination, First Edition. Philip Jevon, Elliot Epstein, Sarah Mensforth, and Caroline MacMahon.
© 2020 John Wiley & Sons Ltd. Published 2020 by John Wiley & Sons Ltd.
Companion website: www.wiley.com/go/jevon/medicalstudent

Cranial nerve I (olfactory)

- Simply ask about alterations in sense of smell, or test one nostril at a time with vials of strong smelling substances such as mint, coffee, or lemon

Cranial nerve II (optic): Four aspects to test

Use the mnemonic AFRO (acuity, fields, reflexes, ophthalmoscopy) to help remember the four aspects to test.

- *Acuity*
  - Using a Snellen chart, test one eye at a time, with and without normal vision aids (glasses, contact lenses). If a Snellen chart is not available, you can ask the patient to read some small print – your hospital badge, the hospital menu, or a line from the newspaper
  - Assess colour vision using Ishihara plates
- *Fields*
  - Test optic fields using the direct confrontation technique. The patient should focus on your nose while you test their peripheral vision. Ensure you test all four quadrants of both eyes, comparing their fields with your own as 'the normal'

 Common misinterpretations and pitfalls

Do not rush, as you may miss subtle defects, and there probably will not be time to repeat the test. When performing this technique, move your finger from the outermost part of the quadrant to the innermost *slowly*, asking regularly 'can you see my fingertip/the hat pin?'

  - Test for visual inattention. Ask the patient to point to which finger is moving whilst they focus on your nose. The patient should be able to detect movement in their peripheral vision on the right and left simultaneously (Figure 5.1)
- *Reflexes*
  - Test the accommodation reflex. Ask the patient to focus on the furthest point the room will allow, then look at your finger, which should be about 10 cm from their nose. Observe for pupil convergence and constriction on near vision
  - Test pupillary light reflexes, direct and consensual. The pupil will constrict when light is applied (direct) and the left pupil should constrict when light is applied to the right, and vice versa

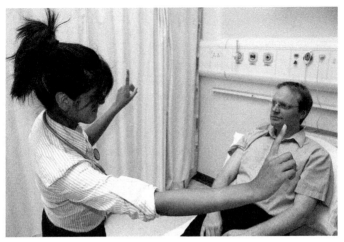

Figure 5.1 Testing for visual inattention.

- *Ophthalmoscopy*
  - Perform fundoscopy

Cranial nerves III (oculomotor), IV (trochlear), and VI (abducens)

- Cranial nerves III, IV, and VI are tested simultaneously, asking the patient to follow your finger as you draw an H shape. CNIII is responsible for all movements apart from intorsion and some depression (CNIV) and lateral movement (CNVI)
- Ask the patient if they have any diplopia during the test, and observe at the extremes of motion for nystagmus

Cranial nerve V (trigeminal)

- *Sensory component*
  - Test facial sensation in the ophthalmic (V1), maxillary (V2), and mandibular (V3) divisions (see Chapter 6 for assessment of sensation)
- *Motor component*
  - Assess power in the masseter, temporalis, and lateral pterygoid muscles
- *Reflex component*
  - Jaw jerk (afferent and efferent limb)
  - Corneal reflex (afferent limb only) – these are not routinely performed

Cranial nerve VII (facial)

- *Sensory component*
  - Ask about changes in taste sense – nerve supplies taste sensation to the anterior two-thirds of the tongue
- *Motor component – muscles of facial expression*
  - Ask the patient to:
    - Raise their eyebrows (frontalis)
    - Close their eyes tightly against resistance (orbicularis oculi)
    - Puff out their cheeks (buccinator)
    - Pout their lips (orbicularis oris)
    - Grimace/show their teeth (platysma)
- *Reflex component*
  - Efferent limb of the corneal reflex

NB An upper motor neuron lesion of CNVII spares the forehead. Bell's palsy is a lower motor neuron lesion, therefore there is unilateral facial droop including of the forehead.

Cranial nerve VIII (vestibular)

- Ask about alteration in sensation of hearing
- Perform the Rinne and Weber tests to discern between sensorineural or conductive deafness (Box 5.1)

Box 5.1 Rinne's and Weber's tests	
Normal or positive Rinne's test	Air conduction is better than bony conduction
Abnormal or negative Rinne's test	Bone conduction is better than air conduction in *conductive deafness*
Normal Weber's test	Sensation transmits equally to both ears
Abnormal Weber's test	Sensation transmits better to the affected ear in *conductive deafness*
Abnormal Weber's test	Sensation transmits better to the normal ear in *sensorineural deafness*

Cranial nerve IX (glossopharyngeal)

- *Sensory component*
  - Ask about altered taste sensation – nerve supplies taste sensation to the posterior one-third of the tongue
  - Gag reflex is not routinely tested – supplies sensation to the pharynx
- *Motor component*
  - Ask the patient to say 'Aaaaah!' and observe for symmetrical palatal elevation – contributes to elevation of the pharynx
  - Observe for a hoarse voice – contributes to innervations of the larynx
- *Reflex component*
  - Afferent limb for gag reflex

Cranial nerve X (vagus)

- Ask the patient to say 'Aaaaah!' and observe for symmetrical palatal elevation and hoarse voice – contributes to musculature of the pharynx and larynx

Cranial nerve XI (accessory)

- Ask the patient to elevate their shoulders against resistance – this tests the power of the trapezius muscle
- Ask the patient to turn their head into resistance provided by your hand on their chin – this tests the power of sternocleidomastoid muscle (Figure 5.2)

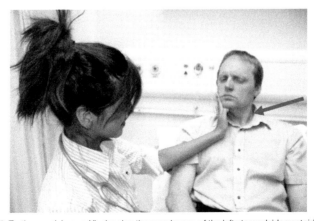

Figure 5.2 Testing cranial nerve XI: showing the prominence of the left sternocleidomastoid as the patient turns against resistance.

Cranial nerve XII (hypoglossal)

- Ask the patient to poke out their tongue. Observe for fasciculations and deviation of the tongue to one side

To complete the examination

- Offer to perform a full neurological examination
- Thank the patient
- Ensure the patient is covered up and comfortable

OSCE Key Learning Points

Neurological system, cranial nerves: example presentation

✔ This 68-year-old lady has presented with blurred vision. I examined her cranial nerves. Cranial nerves I and II appeared intact, though I would need to use a Snellen chart to formally assess visual acuity, and use an ophthalmoscope to perform fundoscopy.

✔ On assessment of eye movements, cranial nerves III, IV, and VI, I identified that she has diplopia and that the diplopia is worse looking to the left. The eye movements are normal apart from that the left eye does not abduct, indicating a left 6th cranial nerve palsy.

✔ There is no nystagmus. Cranial nerves V, VII, VII, IX, X, XI, and XII are intact and both the Rinne's and Weber's tests were normal.

6 Examination of the neurological system – upper limb

OSCE Key Learning Points

✔ Remember to spend time inspecting from the end of the bed

 NB Inspection, tone, power, coordination, reflexes, and sensation.

Preparation

- *Cross infection*: wash and dry hands, bare below the elbow
- *Introductions*: yourself and the task; confirm patient's name and age
- *Consent*: to the procedure
- *Pain*: is the patient in pain
- *Privacy*: ensure privacy, e.g. curtains drawn around bed
- *Position*: seated or on a couch/bed
- *Exposure*: both arms

End of bed inspection

- *Environment*: wheelchair, crutches, frame, orthopaedic shoes
- *Patient*: positioning (e.g. pillow under one arm, leaning to one side), facial features or asymmetry, hearing aids
- *Arms*: muscle bulk, muscle wasting, asymmetry, deformity, resting tremor, scars, fasciculations

 NB Before you touch the patient, ask again about pain.

Medical Student Survival Skills: Clinical Examination, First Edition. Philip Jevon, Elliot Epstein, Sarah Mensforth, and Caroline MacMahon.
© 2020 John Wiley & Sons Ltd. Published 2020 by John Wiley & Sons Ltd.
Companion website: www.wiley.com/go/jevon/medicalstudent

Tone

- Enquire about arthritis or joint pains before performing the movements
- Assess for decreased or increased tone (cogwheel or lead pipe stiffness or spasticity)
- Compare right and left for each movement:
  - Flex and extend at the wrist
  - Flex and extend and supinate at the elbow
  - Abduct and/or circumduct the shoulder

Power

- Test extrapyramidal drift (Figure 6.1). This serves well as a screening test for power in the arms, as well as indicating an upper motor neuron (UMN) lesion on the side that drifts or pronates
- Use Medical Research Council (MRC) grading (Box 6.1) (score 0–5) to describe and compare the right and left sides

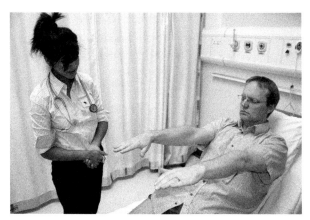

Figure 6.1 Normal position testing for extrapyramidal drift.

Box 6.1 MRC muscle power grading

Grade 5   Normal strength against resistance
Grade 4   Reduced but effective strength against resistance
Grade 3   No strength against resistance, but can move against gravity
Grade 2   Muscle can move the joint if gravity removed
Grade 1   A flicker of movement only
Grade 0   No movement observed

- Test power in
  - *Shoulders*: adduction (testing C6) and abduction (testing C5)
  - *Elbows*: flexion (testing C5, C6) and extension (testing C7, C8)
  - *Wrists*: flexion (testing C6, C7, C8, and median nerve) and extension (testing C6, C7, C8, and radial nerve)
  - *Hands*: finger grip, abduction and adduction of fingers and thumb, and thumb opposition (see Chapter 8 for details)

OSCE Key Learning Points

Which nerves supply the each of the small muscles of the hand?

✔ All are supplied by the ulnar nerve apart from the **LOAF** muscles: the **l**ateral two **l**umbricals, **o**pponens pollicis, **a**bductor pollicis brevis, and **f**lexor pollicis brevis

Coordination

- Perform the finger–nose test to assess for intention tremor and past pointing
- Perform clapping and alternating movements of the pronator/supinator to assess for dysdiadochokinesia

Reflexes

- Compare the right and left for each reflex
- Perform the reflex twice. If not elicited, perform a 'reinforcement' manoeuvre such as asking the patient to clench the jaw

Common misinterpretations and pitfalls

- The patient must be *completely* relaxed; the more relaxed the patient is the better the result
- The patient must clench their jaw at the same time as you strike with the tendon hammer to do the reflex. Try counting 1...2...3 clench!

- *Supinator reflex* – C5, C6 (Figure 6.2): locate the brachioradialis tendon at the wrist. Press your fingers down over this and strike your fingers with the tendon hammer. Observe for supination and slight wrist extension
- *Biceps reflex* – C5, C6 (Figure 6.3): flex the patient's elbow to roughly 90°. Press your thumb across the biceps tendon and strike your thumb with the tendon hammer. Observe for contraction of the biceps muscle or flexion of the elbow
- *Triceps reflex* – C7, C8 (Figure 6.4): support the arm so the elbow is flexed 90° or more. Locate the triceps tendon. Strike the tendon directly and watch for contraction of the triceps muscle

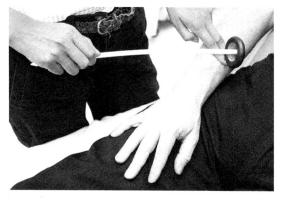

Figure 6.2 Supinator reflex technique.

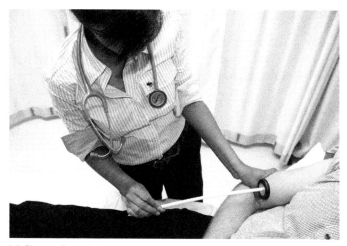

Figure 6.3 Biceps reflex technique.

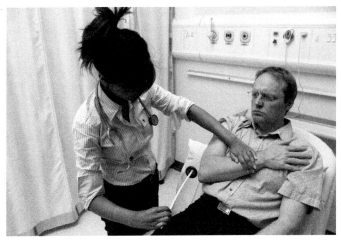

Figure 6.4 Triceps reflex technique.

Sensation

Testing should be performed in each dermatome (Figure 6.5). The patient is usually asked to close their eyes for assessment of fine touch, vibration, and proprioception; however this might induce anxiety for the assessment of sharp touch.

- *Fine touch*
  - Using a neurofilament or the tip of a cotton wool strand, lightly touch the skin (Figure 6.6). Demonstrate the sensation centrally (on the chest) as a reference point
  - Compare each dermatome right and left, and ask if the sensation is reduced or the same on both sides

 Common misinterpretations and pitfalls

Avoid applying *any* pressure when testing fine touch, as this sensation tests other nerve tracts.

- *Sharp touch*: repeat the process as above with a neurotip
- *Temperature*: is not often done, due to equipment limitations
- *Vibration*: test with a 128 Hz tuning fork
  - Demonstrate the sensation centrally (on the chest) as a reference point
  - Test vibration sense on the index fingertip

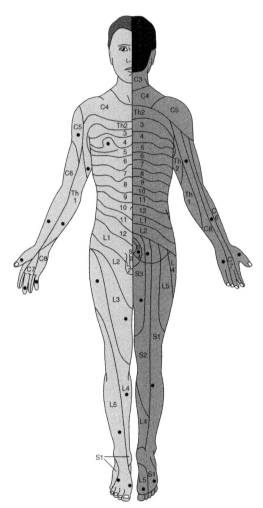

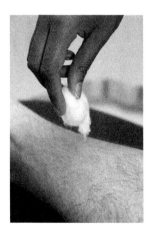

Figure 6.5 Dermatones. Source: Jevon, P. (2009). Clinical
Examination Skills. Oxford: Wiley Blackwell. Reproduced with
permission of Wiley.

Figure 6.6 Testing a dermatome.

- If there is no sensation, progress proximally to the first metacarpophalangeal joint, then the wrist joint, then the elbow, etc.
- Compare right to left, and ask if the sensation is reduced or the same on both sides

OSCE Key Learning Points

✔ Ensure that the patient tells you if they feel the *vibration* of the tuning fork, not the cold metal or pressure

- *Proprioception*
  - Isolate the distal interphalangeal joint of the index finger
  - Demonstrate the upwards and downwards position
  - Flex and extend the distal phalanx, asking the patient to tell you the position, with their eyes closed
  - If proprioception is impaired, isolate a more proximal joint (wrist, then elbow, etc.)

 NB Take care not to hold the dorsum or plantar aspect of the finger, as the pressure can give the patient clues as to the position of the joint.

To complete the examination

- Assess gait
- Examine the cranial nerves and lower limbs
- Thank the patient
- Ensure the patient is covered up and comfortable

OSCE Key Learning Points

Neurological system, upper limb: example presentation

✔ I examined this elderly lady's arms. There is nothing to note around the bed. On inspection of the arms, there were no fasiculations, muscle wasting, or scars. There was a resting tremor of the right hand, which was pill rolling. On assessment of tone, the right arm had increased tone with cogwheel rigidity.

✔ The power, coordination, and reflexes were intact. The tremor disappears when she uses the arm. Sensation was normal. This lady has a resting tremor, therefore I demonstrated other features of Parkinsonism: a shuffling gait; micrographia; and a quiet, monotonous speaking voice.

Examination of the neurological system – lower limb

7

NB Inspection including gait, tone, power, coordination, reflexes, and sensation.

Preparation

- *Cross infection*: wash and dry hands, bare below the elbow
- *Introductions*: yourself and the task; confirm patient's name and age
- *Consent*: to the procedure
- *Pain*: is the patient in pain
- *Privacy*: ensure privacy, e.g. curtains drawn around bed
- *Position*: on the bed at 45° – if this is not possible, report that back to the observer.
- *Exposure*: both legs

End of bed inspection

- *Environment*: wheelchair, crutches, frame, orthopaedic shoes, white cane of visually impaired person

Medical Student Survival Skills: Clinical Examination, First Edition. Philip Jevon, Elliot Epstein, Sarah Mensforth, and Caroline MacMahon.
© 2020 John Wiley & Sons Ltd. Published 2020 by John Wiley & Sons Ltd.
Companion website: www.wiley.com/go/jevon/medicalstudent

- *Patient*: positioning (e.g. pillow under one arm, leaning to one side), facial features or asymmetry, hearing aids
- *Legs*: muscle bulk, muscle wasting, asymmetry, deformity, resting tremor, scars, and fasciculations

 NB Before you touch the patient, ask again about pain.

Tone

- Check about arthritis or joint pains before performing the movements
- Assess for decreased or increased tone, and compare right and left
  - With the legs relaxed, gently roll medially and laterally (Figure 7.1)
  - Place your hand under the knee and sharply lift the knee a few centimetres from the bed, while observing the foot – it should not leave contact with the couch (Figure 7.2)
  - Check for ankle clonus – flex the knee, relax the ankle, then sharply dorsiflex the ankle – watch for several beats of plantar flexion

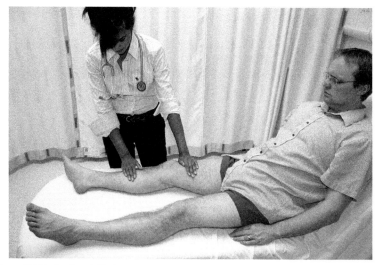

Figure 7.1 Testing tone in the leg.

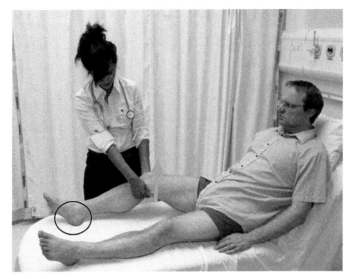

Figure 7.2 Testing tone in the knee.

Power

Use Medical Research Council (MRC) grading to describe, comparing right and left (see Box 6.1). Test power in:

- Hips – flexion (testing L2, L3), extension (L4, L5), adduction (L2, L3, L4), and abduction (L4, L5, S1)
- Knees – flexion (testing L5, S1) and extension (L3, L4)
- Ankles – dorsiflexion (testing L4, L5) and plantar flexion (S1,S2)
- Great toe – flexion (testing S1, S2) and extension (L5, S1)

OSCE Key Learning Points

Causes of reduced power

✔ Symmetrical upper motor neuron (UMN) lesion – spinal cord lesion

✔ Symmetrical lower motor neuron (LMN) lesion – peripheral neuropathy (motor)

✔ Asymmetrical UMN lesion – stroke

✔ Asymmetrical LMN lesion – single nerve palsy

NB Multiple sclerosis and motor neuron disease can cause both UMN and LMN lesions.

Coordination

- Assessment of gait – at the start or the end of the examination
- Perform heel–shin test. Ask the patient to place their left heel to their right knee and hover the heel distally towards their foot and back up to the knee (Figure 7.3)

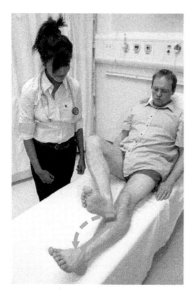

Figure 7.3 Coordination testing in the leg.

Reflexes

- Compare right and left for each reflex
- Perform the reflex twice. If not elicited, perform a 'reinforcement' manoeuvre such as asking the patient to clench the jaw, or clench their hands together

 NB Do not forget to assess gait! You should recognise Parkinsonian, hemiparetic/plegic, scissoring, antalgic, high stepping and ataxic gaits.

- *Knee reflex* – L3, L4 (Figure 7.4): support the knee in slight flexion. Locate the patellar tendon at the knee. Strike the tendon with the hammer. Observe for quadriceps contraction
- *Ankle reflex* – S1, S2: flex the knee and relax laterally. Dorsiflex the ankle and strike the tendon with the hammer. Observe for plantarflexion of the foot
- *Plantar reflex* – L5, S1: using an orange stick, apply pressure in a sweeping motion from proximal to distal down the lateral aspect of the sole of the foot, continuing medially across the metatarsal heads. Observe for extension of the great toe – this is abnormal

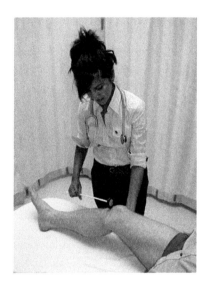

Figure 7.4 Technique for the knee reflex.

Sensation

Testing should be performed in each dermatome, and is described fully in Chapter 6.

- *Fine touch*
  - Using a neurofilament, demonstrate on the chest before assessing dermatomes. Compare right to left

---

OSCE Key Learning Points

✔ Be clear with your instructions: 'I am going to touch your skin with this (neurotip/cotton wool) I want you to say "Yes" when you feel it. Tell me if it's the same or different on the left and right'

- *Sharp touch*: repeat the process as above with a neurotip
- *Temperature*: is not often done, due to equipment limitations
- *Vibration*: test with a 128 Hz tuning fork
  - Demonstrate the sensation on the chest, then begin by assessing vibration sense in the tip of the great toe. If there is no sensation move to the lateral malleolus of the ankle, and then the patella
  - Compare right to left, and ask if the sensation is reduced or the same on both sides

OSCE Key Learning Points

✔ Vibration and fine touch are carried in the dorsal columns tract. Pain and temperature are carried in the spinothalamic tract. It is possible therefore to have intact pain sense and impaired vibration sense in the same area

- *Proprioception*
  - Isolate the interphalangeal joint of the great toe
  - Demonstrate the upwards and downwards position
  - Flex and extend the distal phalanx, asking the patient to tell you the position, with their eyes closed
  - If proprioception is impaired, isolate a more proximal joint (ankle then knee, etc.)

 Common misinterpretations and pitfalls

Neurological examination is often dreaded by medical students and there is a tendency to 'go through the routine' whilst not picking up on the signs. Remember to observe carefully, think as you go along:
- Is that an UMN sign or a LMN sign?
- If you find an intention tremor think about what other cerebellar signs you can demonstrate

To complete the examination

- Assess gait
- Examine the cranial nerves and upper limb
- Thank the patient
- Ensure the patient is covered up and comfortable

OSCE Key Learning Points

Neurological system, lower limb: example presentation

✔ I examined this gentleman's lower limbs. On inspection round the bed, I noted a walking stick, and orthopaedic shoes. On inspection, there were no obvious scars, swelling, or deformities; however there were bilateral trophic changes and a callus under the metatarsal heads on the left foot.

✔ Tone, power, reflexes, and coordination were normal. There was no light touch sensation in the toes bilaterally, and reduced sensation in the feet. The sensation was normal at the mid shin. This was the same in modalities of vibration, proprioception, and sharp touch. This suggests a sensory peripheral neuropathy. To conclude the examination I would examine the arms for similar features.

8 Examination of musculoskeletal system – the hands

 NB Follow the usual routine for musculoskeletal examinations; look, feel, move, and neurovascular status, followed by special tests.

Preparation

- *Cross infection*: wash and dry hands, bare below the elbow
- *Introductions*: yourself and the task; confirm patient's name and age
- *Consent*: to the procedure
- *Pain*: is the patient in pain
- *Privacy*: ensure privacy, e.g. curtains drawn around bed
- *Position*: ideally sitting in a chair, with hands positioned comfortably on a pillow and table
- *Exposure*: expose from the forearm down. Ideally, ask the patient to unbutton their sleeves and roll them up during the examination to demonstrate their functional status

End of bed inspection

- *Environment*: walking aids, beakers or cups, crosswords and pens, cutlery, inhalers, screw top bottles – all give you an idea about the function of their hands
- *Patient*: mobility, posture (kyphosis, neck brace)

Medical Student Survival Skills: Clinical Examination, First Edition. Philip Jevon, Elliot Epstein, Sarah Mensforth, and Caroline MacMahon.
© 2020 John Wiley & Sons Ltd. Published 2020 by John Wiley & Sons Ltd.
Companion website: www.wiley.com/go/jevon/medicalstudent

Inspection

- *Inspect the dorsal side*
  - Skin for colour (red/blue), psoriatic plaques, scars, bruising, rashes, telangietasia (Figure 8.1), sclerodactyly (Figure 8.2), fingertip infarcts, gouty tophi (Figure 8.3)
  - Joints for swelling (synovitis, Heberden's and Bouchard's nodes), deformities (ulnar deviation, Z thumb, swan neck, boutonniere deformity), subluxation and dislocations, rheumatoid nodules
  - Nails for infarcts, onycholysis, pitting, hyperkeratosis, Beau's lines, clubbing, leuchonychia, koilonychia
  - Muscles for interossei wasting
- *Inspect the palmar side*
  - Skin changes as above
  - Muscles for hypothenar and thenar eminence wasting
- *Hand and fingers*
  - Size/shape
  - Large, square, and doughy? – acromegaly
  - Arachnodactyly? Hypermobile joints? – Marfan's syndrome
- *Elbows*
  - Skin plaques, rashes, rheumatoid nodules, synovitis
- *Face*
  - Examine posterior to ears and the hairline for skin psoriatic plaques, look for skin tightening (scleroderma), acromegaly features, butterfly rash of systemic lupus erythematosus (SLE), and ears for gouty tophi

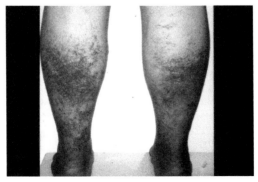

Figure 8.1 Telangietasia.

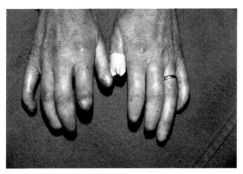

Figure 8.2 Sclerodactyly.

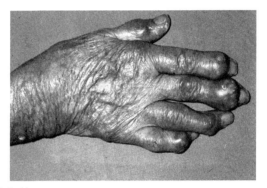

Figure 8.3 Gouty tophi.

 Common misinterpretations and pitfalls

Inspection will provide you with a huge amount of information. Ensure you complete 'inspection' before moving on to 'feel'.

Feel

Incorporate *vascular status* here.
- Assess temperature on both sides simultaneously with the backs of your hands
- Assess capillary refill time
- Assess radial pulse

- Palpate each joint starting with the distal interphalangeals (DIPs) and then proximal interphalangeals (PIPs) using the index finger and thumb (Figure 8.4). Palpate the metacarpophalangeals (MCPs) and wrist supporting the joint with your fingers underneath and using your thumbs to palpate
  - Note the presence of pain, swelling, osteophytes, and crepitus
  - Look at the patient's face whilst examining to assess for pain
- Feel for tendon thickening – Dupuytren's contracture

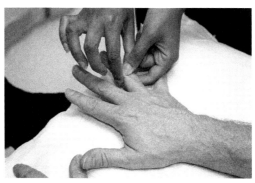

Figure 8.4 Correct technique for palpating the DIPs and PIPs.

OSCE Key Learning Points

Common features of rheumatoid arthritis in the hands

✔ Z thumb, swan neck, boutonniere, ulnar deviation, subluxation of the MCPs, nodules, bruising, scars from joint replacements, boggy synovitis

✔ If there is active inflammation, the joint may be hot and erythematous

Move

Demonstrate movements to show range of movement (ROM) and power of the muscles. Compare right and left, testing each side simultaneously.

- *Wrist*
  - Demonstrate ROM with the 'prayer' (Figure 8.5) and 'inverse prayer' (Figure 8.6) movements
  - Demonstrate radial nerve function by asking the patient to extend the wrist against resistance (Figure 8.7). This test should be done with the patient's arm on their knee for stability

- *Fingers*
  - Demonstrate ROM and power of:
    - Finger flexion with hand gripping your index finger – try to pull your fingers away
    - Abduction of fingers

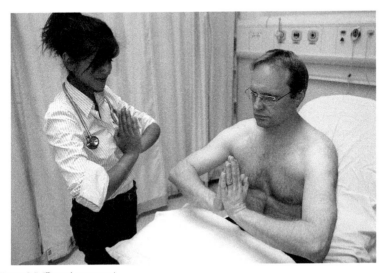

Figure 8.5 'Prayer' movement.

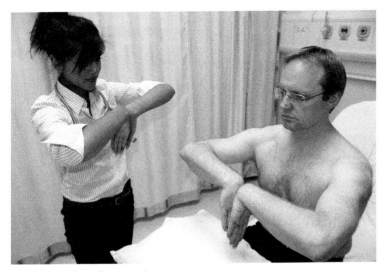

Figure 8.6 Inverse 'prayer' movement.

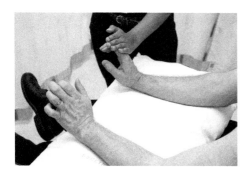

Figure 8.7 Testing wrist extension.

 NB When testing finger abduction, *compare like for like* with your index and little finger, not the thumb and index finger.

- ■ Adduction of fingers – test by asking the patient to grip a piece of paper between their index and middle fingers and try to pull this from them using your index and middle fingers (Figure 8.8)
- – Demonstrate the function of the ulnar nerve by performing Froment's test (Figure 8.9): ask the patient to grasp a piece of paper between their thumb and index finger, and resist this being pulled away. If they flex their thumb in an effort to keep the paper, this shows weakness of the adductor pollicis (innervated by the ulnar nerve)
- ● *Thumb*
  - – Demonstrate opposition of finger and thumb to make a pincer
  - – Demonstrate thumb abduction against resistance to test median nerve function
- ● *Function*
  - – Ask the patient to demonstrate holding a pen, writing, picking up a small object, buttoning up clothing, holding cutlery, etc.

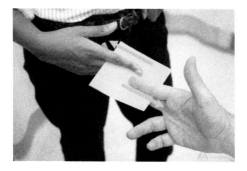

Figure 8.8 Testing strength of adduction.

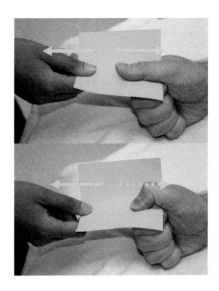

Figure 8.9 Froment's test.

Sensation

For a description of detailed testing see Chapter 6. Demonstrate the sensory areas for the median, ulnar, and radial nerves.

To complete the examination

- Offer to examine the feet and other joints
- If you find features of rheumatoid, Marfan's, acromegaly, etc. offer to examine for extra-articular features
- Thank the patient
- Ensure patient is covered up and comfortable

OSCE Key Learning Points

Musculoskeletal system, the hands: example presentation

✔ On examination round the bed I can see that this lady has a walking stick. On inspection of her hands, I can see that she has dorsal muscle wasting, and joint swelling in the DIPs and PIPs. There are no nail changes and no skin changes. On palpation, the DIPs and PIPs are non-tender and have bony swelling, consistent with Heberden's and Bouchard's nodes.

✔ On examination of movements, the wrist, finger, and thumb were tested. All movements were full, with good power. Motor and sensory function of the radial, ulnar, and median nerves were intact, and the hands were warm with good radial pulses. To complete the examination I would examine the joints of the lower limbs. I suspect that this lady has osteoarthritis.

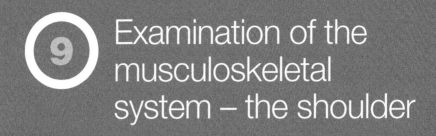

Examination of the musculoskeletal system – the shoulder

OSCE Key Learning Points

✔ Remember to spend time inspecting from the end of the bed

NB Follow the usual routine for musculoskeletal examinations; look, feel, move, and neurovascular status, followed by special tests.

Preparation

- *Cross infection*: wash and dry hands, bare below the elbow
- *Introductions*: yourself and the task; confirm patient's name and age
- *Consent*: to the procedure
- *Pain*: is the patient in pain
- *Privacy*: ensure privacy, e.g. curtains drawn around bed
- *Position*: the patient should ideally be standing
- *Exposure*: from the waist up (shirt off)

End of bed inspection

- *Environment*: slings, medication
- *Patient*: pain, distress, position, general health

NB Do not forget to examine the good joint first, and compare both sides throughout your examination.

Medical Student Survival Skills: Clinical Examination, First Edition. Philip Jevon, Elliot Epstein, Sarah Mensforth, and Caroline MacMahon.
© 2020 John Wiley & Sons Ltd. Published 2020 by John Wiley & Sons Ltd.
Companion website: www.wiley.com/go/jevon/medicalstudent

OSCE Key Learning Points

✔ Ask the patient to tell you if they feel pain at any time

OSCE Key Learning Points

Differential diagnoses of a painful shoulder include

✔ Soft tissue: tendonitis (supraspinatus, long head of biceps), bursitis, nerve entrapment, adhesive capsulitis (Box 9.1), gout

✔ Joint: dislocation, subluxation, arthritis (glenohumeral or acromioclavicular)

✔ Bone: fracture, infection, neoplasm, avascular necrosis

✔ Referred pain: cervical spine pathology, cardiac pain, apical lung tumours

Box 9.1 Adhesive capsulitis

Adhesive capsulitis or frozen shoulder is an idiopathic condition causing globally reduced movement of the glenohumeral joint. It is described in three stages: the painful stage, the adhesive stage, and the recovery stage. It is most common in patients in their 50s and 60s, and is more common in women. Clinical examination reveals loss of passive and active movement in all planes of the shoulder. Management includes physiotherapy, and intra-articular glucocorticoid injections, although spontaneous recovery is common.

Inspection

Surface anatomy of the shoulder is shown in Figure 9.1. Inspect from the front, side, and back, looking for:

- Scars: look closely for small scars of previous arthroscopy
- Swelling
- Erythema: inflammation, e.g. infection or rheumatoid arthritis
- Deformity: loss of contour or symmetry of the shoulders
- Muscle wasting: of the deltoid, biceps, or pectoralis major

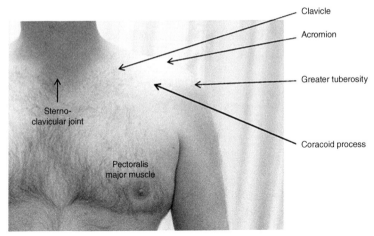

Clavicle

Acromion

Greater tuberosity

Sterno-
clavicular joint

Coracoid process

Pectoralis
major muscle

Figure 9.1 Surface anatomy of the shoulder.

OSCE Key Learning Points

Glenohumeral dislocation

✔ *Anterior dislocation* (95% of glenohumeral dislocations): abduction and external rotation of the shoulder

✔ Posterior dislocation (rare): can occur during seizures

✔ Clinical features: flattened shoulder contour, prominent humeral head, and arm in abduction and internal rotation

Feel

- Temperature: assess with the back of your hand. Assess both sides together to detect any difference
- Systematically palpate the following landmarks, feeling for tenderness, deformity, and swelling:
  - Sternoclavicular joint (SCJ)
  - Clavicle
  - Acromioclavicular joint (ACJ)
  - Glenohumeral joint line
  - Spine of scapula
  - Medial border of scapula
- Test for numbness of the 'badge area' (axillary nerve injury)

OSCE Key Learning Points

✔ The axillary nerve (C5, C6) is easily damaged by dislocation of the shoulder

✔ This nerve supplies the deltoid and teres minor muscles, therefore injury causes loss of shoulder abduction and external rotation

Move

Observe passive then active movement. Observe and report the degree of flexion and extension, and observe for symmetry of movement.

- Ask the patient to put their hands behind their head. This examines abduction and external rotation and is a good screening test of active shoulder movement

- *Flexion/extension*: ask the patient to extend both arms in front of them to a vertical position, then back down. Observe the movement in the glenohumeral joint initially, followed by elevation of the scapula to achieve full flexion

- *Abduction*: the patient brings both arms straight out to the side, thumbs forward and elbows extended, again reaching a vertical position. Observe movement of the glenohumeral joint and scapula. If there is pain, note the degree of abduction at which it occurs (see box on painful arc syndrome)

- *Internal rotation*: ask the patient to place their hand as far up their back as they can. Compare the right and left sides

- *External rotation*: with elbows flexed and arms tucked into the side, the patient opens their forearms outwards. This is typically reduced in adhesive capsulitis

- *Test* muscle power against resistance

NB Abduction of the shoulder is produced by movement of the following:

0–30°: supraspinatus

30–90°: deltoid

90–180°: scapula

OSCE Key Learning Points

Painful arc syndrome

✔ Pain occurring at different degrees of abduction can point towards the underlying pathology

✔ An important feature is absence of pain while moving through the rest of the arc

✔ 60–120°: supraspinatus tendonitis

✔ 140–180°: ACJ osteoarthritis

The rotator cuff muscles

Table 9.1 gives details of the four rotator cuff muscles.

Table 9.1 Features of the rotator cuff muscles

	Supraspinatus	Infraspinatus	Teres minor	Subscapularis
Origin	Supraspinous fossa of scapula	Infraspinous fossa of scapula	Lateral border of scapula	Subscapular fossa of scapula
Insertion	Greater tubercle of humerus (superior facet)	Greater tubercle of humerus (middle facet)	Greater tubercle of humerus (inferior facet)	Lesser tubercle of humerus
Action	Abduction (first 30°)	External rotation	External rotation	Internal rotation
Innervation	Suprascapular nerve (C5, C6)	Subscapular nerve (C5, C6)	Axillary nerve (C5, C6)	Subscapular nerve (C5, C6)
Test by	Internally rotate arm, elbow extended Flex and abduct shoulder to 30° Ask patient to push up against resistance	Resisted external rotation with elbows flexed to 90° and tucked into sides		Hand behind back, pushing out against resistance

OSCE Key Learning Points

Impingement syndrome

✔ This is mechanical compression of the rotator cuff under the acromion

✔ The rotator cuff muscles run in a narrow space between the acromion process of the scapula and the head of the humerus, therefore this clinical picture may be produced by pathology that reduces this space

✔ Causes include supraspinatus tendonitis, long head of biceps tendonitis, ACJ arthritis, and subacromial bursitis

Special tests

- *Impingement*:
  - Hawkin's test (Figure 9.2): with one hand on the patient's elbow and the other on their wrist, flex the elbow to 90° while placing the shoulder in a position of 80° of flexion and 30° abduction. While supporting the elbow, apply gentle downwards pressure to the wrist, internally rotating the shoulder. This action reduces the space under the ACJ, and will produce pain in a patient with impingement syndrome
- Other tests of impingement include the scarf test
- *Rotator cuff muscles*: see Table 9.1
- *Winged scapula*: ask the patient to push against a wall, with the shoulder flexed and elbows extended. Injury to the long thoracic nerve of Bell (C5–C7) may cause winging of the scapula due to weakness of serratus anterior

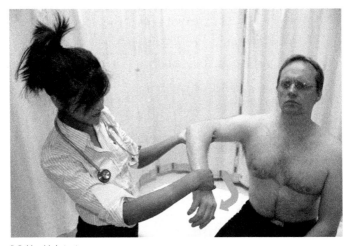

Figure 9.2 Hawkin's test.

To complete the examination

- Complete neurovascular status of the upper limbs
- Check for lymphadenopathy
- Observe function (by observing them replace their shirt)
- Offer to examine the joint above (cervical spine) and below (elbow)
- Thank the patient
- Ensure the patient is covered up and comfortable

OSCE Key Learning Points

Musculoskeletal system, the shoulder: example presentation

✔ This is Mr Davis, a 35-year-old gentleman who presents with pain in his left shoulder. On general examination he is alert and orientated and comfortable at rest, and in good general health with a normal body mass index.

✔ On inspection of the shoulder, there were no scars, swelling, erythema, or obvious asymmetry. On palpation, there was tenderness of the acromioclavicular joint. Full range of movement was demonstrated in all planes, but there was pain on abduction of the left shoulder at a position of 90–110°. Examination of the rotator cuff revealed weakness of abduction with an internally rotated shoulder, and Hawkin's impingement test was positive.

✔ In summary, this gentleman displays clinical signs consistent with impingement syndrome due to supraspinatus tendonitis.

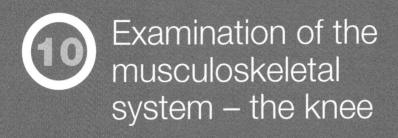

10 Examination of the musculoskeletal system – the knee

OSCE Key Learning Points

✔ Remember to spend time inspecting from the end of the bed

NB Follow the usual routine for musculoskeletal examinations; look, feel, move, and neurovascular status, followed by special tests.

Preparation

- *Cross infection*: wash and dry hands, bare below the elbow
- *Introductions*: yourself and the task; confirm patient's name and age
- *Consent*: to the procedure
- *Pain*: is the patient in pain
- *Privacy*: ensure privacy, e.g. curtains drawn around bed
- *Position*: standing initially, then on the bed at 45° – if this is not possible, report that back to the observer.
- *Exposure*: from the waist down, to underwear, feet exposed

End of bed inspection

- *Environment*: walking aids, orthopaedic shoes
- *Patient*: pain, distress, position, general health

Medical Student Survival Skills: Clinical Examination, First Edition. Philip Jevon, Elliot Epstein, Sarah Mensforth, and Caroline MacMahon.
© 2020 John Wiley & Sons Ltd. Published 2020 by John Wiley & Sons Ltd.
Companion website: www.wiley.com/go/jevon/medicalstudent

NB Inspection includes gait, tone, power, coordination, reflexes, and sensation.

 NB Always examine the good joint first. You will be better placed to detect any abnormality if you are familiar with what is normal for that patient. Ligamentous laxity in particular can vary significantly between patients.

OSCE Key Learning Points

Radiographic features of osteoarthritis

✔ Loss of joint space
✔ Subchondral sclerosis
✔ Cysts
✔ Osteophytes

Inspection

Inspect from the front, side and back, with the patient standing, looking for the following:

- Scars: may suggest joint replacement, arthroscopy, or vascular surgery
- Swelling
- Erythema
- Asymmetry
- Deformity
- Muscle wasting

OSCE Key Learning Points

Common deformities of the knee

✔ Valgus: lateral displacement of the distal tibia and fibula
✔ Varus: medial displacement of the distal tibia and fibula
✔ Fixed flexion: patient is unable to fully extend the knee
✔ Osteoarthritis: most common cause of knee deformities

It is helpful to inspect gait at this point, before you ask the patient to lie down.

Feel

At this point ask the patient to move to the couch, and perform the remainder of the examination with them supine. Knowledge of the surface anatomy of the knee is particularly helpful.

- Temperature: assess with the back of your hand. Assess both together to detect any differences
- Effusion: bulge test or patellar tap
- Fixed flexion deformity: place your hand under the knee and ask the patient to push their knee towards the couch, onto your hand. If they cannot do this, there is fixed flexion deformity
- Systematically palpate the following landmarks, feeling for tenderness and swelling:
  - Quadriceps tendon
  - Patellar margins
  - Patellar tendon
  - Joint line (with knee flexed to 30°); tenderness here may indicate meniscal pathology (McMurray's test)
- Side to side movement of the patella
- Perform patella tap test (Figure 10.1)

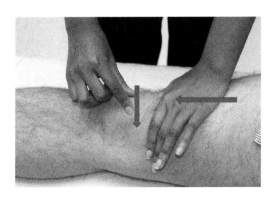

Figure 10.1 Patellar tap test.

NB Increased joint temperature may indicate septic arthritis, inflammatory arthritis, gout, or deep vein thrombosis.

OSCE Key Learning Points

How to examine for effusion by the patellar tap test (Figure 10.1)

✔ Empty the suprapatellar pouch by sweeping the left hand from the mid-thigh to the quadriceps tendon (this needs to be fairly firm)

✔ Keeping the left hand in place, gently press on the anterior surface of the patellar with the right hand. You will feel a tapping if there is effusion

Move

Observe passive then active movement. Observe and report the degree of flexion and extension, in degrees. A normal knee should flex to around 140°.

- Flexion
- Extension
- Hand on knee to detect any crepitus

 NB Mechanism of common ligamentous injuries:

- *Cruciate ligaments*: twisting movements or sudden change of direction, e.g. footballers
- *Medial collateral*: lateral blow to the lateral knee, e.g. car hitting a pedestrian

Special tests

- *Posterior sag sign*: examining for deficiency of the posterior cruciate ligaments. Bend both knees to 90° and inspect carefully from the side. If there is laxity of the posterior cruciate the tibial head will slip posteriorly against the femur, thus giving a sagging appearance
- *Drawer sign* (Figure 10.2): with the knees remaining flexed to 90°, sit at the patient's feet and face towards them. Starting with the unaffected knee, place your hands firmly either side of the superior tibia, and pull forwards. Watch the patient's face to ensure you are not causing them pain. Repeat this on the affected side. Forwards displacement of the tibia relative to the femur indicates insufficiency of the anterior collateral ligament

- *Lachman's test* (Figure 10.3): this is another test of the anterior cruciate ligament (ACL). This is difficult to perform if you have small hands but is often more sensitive than the anterior drawer sign. With the knee flexed slightly to around 20°, place your right hand on the distal femur, above the knee, and your left hand below the knee, holding the proximal tibia. Attempt to slide the tibia forwards relative to the femur. An intact ACL will hold the tibia in place, therefore sliding forward indicates a positive test
- *Collateral ligaments*: hold the lower leg supported along your forearm, and flex the knee to 30°. To test the medial collateral, apply pressure to the lateral side of the knee, applying valgus stress to the knee. The lateral collateral is tested by applying varus stress to the knee, by pushing outwards from the medial side

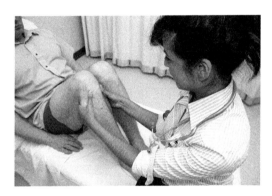

Figure 10.2 Drawer sign.

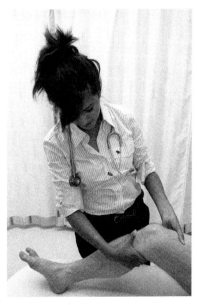

Figure 10.3 Lachman's test.

NB McMurray's test for meniscal injury
The principal of this test is to trap the meniscus between the femoral condyle and the tibia. On the medial side this is achieved by hyperflexion of the knee and adding varus stress while extending the knee, palpating for a click with your left hand over the medial joint line. As you might imagine, this test can be painful for the patient, and in untrained hands it is not very sensitive.

The pivot shift test for ACL injury falls into the same category, and is best avoided in an examination.

Function

- Ask the patient to walk if this has not already been done
- Observe for antalgic gait, stability, foot drop

To complete the examination

- Offer to examine the joint above (hip) and below (ankle)
- Offer to perform a neurovascular examination of the lower limbs
- Thank the patient
- Ensure the patient is covered up and comfortable

OSCE Key Learning Points

Musculosketetal system, the knee: example presentation

✔ This is Mr Jones, a 35-year-old gentleman who presents with pain in his left knee following a sporting injury. On general examination he is alert and orientated and comfortable at rest, and in good general health with normal body mass index.

✔ The knee has a normal appearance on inspection, with no scars, swelling, or muscle wasting. The knee was non-tender to palpation with no clinically apparent effusion. There was full range of active and passive movement. The posterior sag sign was negative, but the drawer test revealed anterior movement of the tibial relative to the femur. This laxity was confirmed with Lachman's test, and could be further examined using the pivot shift test, which I have not performed. Medial and lateral collaterals appeared intact.

✔ In summary, this fit and well 35-year-old man has presented with knee pain, and displays features consistent with injury to the anterior cruciate ligament.

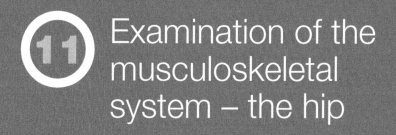

Examination of the musculoskeletal system – the hip

NB Follow the usual routine for musculoskeletal examinations; look, feel, move, and neurovascular status, followed by special tests.

Preparation

- *Cross infection*: wash and dry hands, bare below the elbow
- *Introductions*: yourself and the task; confirm patient's name and age
- *Consent*: to the procedure
- *Pain*: is the patient in pain
- *Privacy*: ensure privacy, e.g. curtains drawn around bed
- *Position*: standing initially, then on the bed at 45° – if this is not possible, report that back to the observer
- *Exposure*: from the waist down, feet exposed

End of bed inspection

- *Environment*: walking aids, orthopaedic shoes
- *Patient*: pain, distress, position, general health

NB Remember to examine the good joint first.

Medical Student Survival Skills: Clinical Examination, First Edition. Philip Jevon, Elliot Epstein, Sarah Mensforth, and Caroline MacMahon.
© 2020 John Wiley & Sons Ltd. Published 2020 by John Wiley & Sons Ltd.
Companion website: www.wiley.com/go/jevon/medicalstudent

OSCE Key Learning Points

✔ During examination, observe the patient's face for pain

Inspection

Inspect from the front (Figure 11.1), side and back, with the patient standing, looking for

- Scars
- Erythema
- Deformity: pelvic tilt or increased lumbar lordosis?
- Gluteal muscle wasting

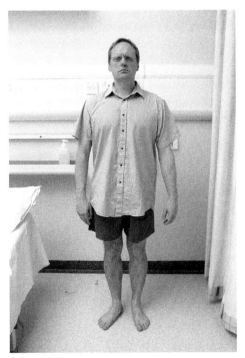

Figure 11.1 Inspect the front.

While the patient is standing, perform the following:

- Trendelenburg's test
- Gait: ask the patient to walk a few metres away from you and back again, watching closely as they walk

OSCE Key Learning Points

Trendelenburg's test (test of hip stability)

✔ If positive it may indicate weakness of the hip abductors

✔ Sit on a chair facing the patient, with their hands on your shoulders

✔ Place one thumb on each anterior superior iliac spine (ASIS). To test the right side, ask the patient to raise the left leg. Dropping of the left hip indicates a positive test

OSCE Key Learning Points

Types of gait

✔ Trendelenburg gait: leaning to one side to correct gluteal weakness

✔ Cerebellar ataxia: unsteady, swinging, wide-based gait

✔ Antalgic gait: reduced pressure placed on the affected side, therefore the stance phase is shortened relative to the swing phase

✔ Parkinsonian: shuffling, slow, with shortened steps

OSCE Key Learning Points

Clinical features of a fractured neck of femur

✔ Shortened leg length

✔ External rotation

✔ Inability to weight bear

- Ask the patient to lie supine on the couch. Observe how easy or difficult this is for them

Feel

- Temperature: assess with the back of your hand. Examine both together to detect any differences
- Systematically palpate the following landmarks, feeling for tenderness and swelling:
  - ASIS
  - Greater trochanter
  - Anterior joint line

- Apparent leg lengths: measure from xiphisternum to medial malleolus
  - Discrepancy indicates fixed adduction deformity
- True leg length
  - Measure from each ASIS to medial malleolus
  - If there is shortening, ask the patient to flex the knees to 90°. By comparing the knee positions, identify whether the shortening is from above or below the knee
- Thomas' test: at rest, a fixed flexion deformity of the hip can be masked by lumbar lordosis. With the patient flat, place one hand under the lumbar spine. To test the left side, lift the patient's right leg by flexion of the hip and knee. This will correct the lordosis of the lumbar spine, confirmed by pressure on your left hand. If a fixed flexion deformity is present, the left knee will lift from the couch. It is important to perform this test before assessing hip movements

 NB Osteoarthritis may cause contractures that limit movement and lead to fixed flexion deformities. The most common of these are fixed flexion (examined by the Thomas test) and fixed adduction (apparent leg shortening).

Move

All movements should be assessed passively, actively, and against resistance. Observe and report the degree of movement in degrees and muscle power according to the Medical Research Council grading system (grades 1–5) (see Chapter 6).

- *Flexion* (normal range 0–130°)
  - Place one hand on the knee and the other on their foot, and flex at the hip
  - Ensure the contralateral hip remains extended (leg lying flat on the couch)
  - While the hip is flexed to 90°, test internal and external rotation
- *Extension* (0–10°)
  - This is examined in a prone position if the patient is able to lie on their front
- *Abduction* (0–45°)
- *Adduction* (0–45°)
  - The foot is crossed over the opposite limb

- *Internal rotation* (0–45°)
  - With the hip and knee both flexed to 90°, place one hand on the knee while the other grips the ankle
  - Produced by lateral movement of the foot with the hip flexed
- *External rotation* (0–30°)
  - Bring the foot medially

To complete the examination

- Offer to examine the joint above and below
- Offer to perform a neurovascular examination of the lower limbs
- Thank the patient and make sure they are comfortable

OSCE Key Learning Points

Musculosketelal system, the hip: example presentation

✔ This is Mrs Smith, an 82-year-old lady who presents with pain of her right hip. On general examination she is alert and orientated and comfortable at rest, with no obvious peripheral stigmata of disease.

✔ On inspection of the hip, there are no visible scars or erythema, though there is some wasting of the quadriceps muscles on the right. On palpation, there was tenderness along the anterior joint line, and the Thomas test was normal showing no fixed flexion deformity. Apparent leg length was 3 cm shorter on the left, though true leg lengths were equal bilaterally, indicating a fixed pelvic tilt towards the right side.

✔ On movement, there was full range of flexion, extension, adduction, and abduction, but internal and external rotation were each limited to 20°.

✔ I would like to complete my examination by performing a full neurological exam of the lower limbs and by examining the spine and the knee.

✔ In summary, this lady shows signs consistent with early osteoarthritis of the hip, which I could investigate further with the use of plain X-ray.

12 Examination of the peripheral arterial system

Preparation

- *Cross infection*: wash and dry hands, bare below the elbow
- *Introductions*: yourself and the task; confirm patient's name and age
- *Consent*: to the procedure
- *Pain*: is the patient in pain
- *Privacy*: ensure privacy, e.g. curtains drawn around bed
- *Position*: ideally supine on a bed
- *Exposure*: from the waist down, underwear on, feet exposed

End of bed inspection

- *Environment*: glyceryl trinitrate (GTN) spray, oxygen, walking aids, evidence of smoking
- *Patient*: breathlessness, distress

 NB Your assessment of the general health of the patient is essential in assessing their fitness for any surgical intervention.

The peripheries

- *Hands*
  - Look for colour (pallor or peripheral cyanosis), tar staining, onycholysis
  - Feel for temperature and capillary refill time (CRT)

Medical Student Survival Skills: Clinical Examination, First Edition. Philip Jevon, Elliot Epstein, Sarah Mensforth, and Caroline MacMahon.
© 2020 John Wiley & Sons Ltd. Published 2020 by John Wiley & Sons Ltd.
Companion website: www.wiley.com/go/jevon/medicalstudent

- – Radial pulse: rate and rhythm
- – Ask for blood pressure
- *Face*
  - – Look for central cyanosis, xanthelasma, corneal arcus
- *Neck*
  - – Carotid pulse
- *Chest*
  - – Sternotomy scar – may indicate a previous coronary artery bypass graft (CABG) or cardiac valve surgery
- *Abdomen*
  - – Palpate for abdominal aortic aneurysm (AAA)

The lower limbs

Inspection

- Scars: vein harvest, endarterectomy, or bypass. Look in the groin and popliteal fossae
- Colour: pallor is characteristic of arterial disease
- Ulcers: look under heel and between toes (Table 12.1)
- Skin: thin and shiny with hair loss is typical of arterial disease
- Muscle atrophy
- Gangrene

Table 12.1 Characteristics of Ulcers

	Arterial	Venous
Position	Feet, heels, toes	Gaiter area
Edges	Regular, 'punched out'	Irregular
Base	Dark colour, typically does not bleed	Granulation tissue
Exudate	Dry	exudative
Pain	Often	Rarely

OSCE Key Learning Points

✔ If a patient has thickened toenails, CRT can be observed by applying pressure to the plantar aspect of the big toe

Palpation

- Temperature (Figure 12.1): may be reduced
- CRT (Figure 12.2): should be <2 seconds. Compare left and right
- Oedema: coexistent venous disease?

Pulses

- *Dorsalis pedis*
  - Lateral to tendon of extensor hallucis longus (Figure 12.3)
- *Posterior tibial*
  - 2 cm inferoposterior to the medial malleolus
- *Popliteal*
  - Should be difficult to palpate, if very obvious consider whether there is an aneurysm
- *Femoral*

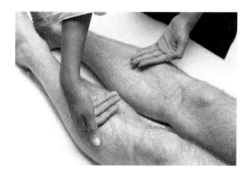

Figure 12.1 Measuring temperature using backs of the hands.

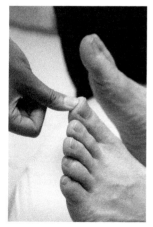

Figure 12.2 Measuring capillary refill time.

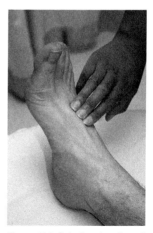

Figure 12.3 Palpating dorsalis pedis.

OSCE Key Learning Points

Features of critical limb ischaemia (the 6 'P's)

✔ Pain

✔ Pallor

✔ Pulselessness

✔ Perishingly cold

✔ Parasthaesia

✔ Paralysis

NB Fontaine classification of peripheral arterial disease:

Stage I: Asymptomatic

Stage II: Intermittent claudication

Stage III: Rest pain

Stage IV: Tissue loss, i.e. necrosis or ulcers

Handheld Doppler ultrasound

This technique is performed in the clinic and is an essential component of your examination (Figure 12.4). You will be expected to use it in an exam so ensure you are comfortable with it. Use whenever you find weak or impalpable pulses.

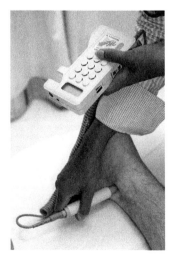

Figure 12.4 Technique for Doppler ultrasound.

NB Doppler ultrasound waveforms provide information about the stenosis of the vessel in question. Elastic recoil in a healthy artery will give a triphasic sound. This becomes lost with increasing atherosclerotic disease, moving to a biphasic and eventually monophasic sound.

Features of embolic versus thrombotic ischaemia

Acute limb ischaemia may be caused by a number of pathologies. If resulting from vascular occlusion, this may be either thrombosis of pre-existing atheroma, or it can be due to emboli from a distant site (Table 12.2). This is an important distinction, as the treatment is different.

Table 12.2 Clinical features of emboli and thrombosis

Clinical features	Embolus	Thrombosis
Severity	Complete (no collaterals)	Incomplete (collaterals)
Onset	Seconds or minutes	Hours or days
Limb affected (leg: arm)	3:1	10:1
Multiple sites	Up to 15%	Rare
Embolic source	Present (usually atrial fibrillation)	Absent
Previous claudication	Absent	Present
Contralateral leg pulses	Present	Absent
Diagnosis	Clinical	Clinical and angiography
Treatment	Embolectomy, warfarin	Medical, angioplasty, bypass

Buerger's test

- Slowly raise one leg upwards (ask about hip pain first!) (Figure 12.5)
- Observe the leg for any colour change, and for venous guttering
- If pallor develops, note the angle at which this occurs (this is called Buerger's angle: smaller indicates more severe disease)
- Lower the leg over the side of the bed
- Observe for reactive hyperaemia

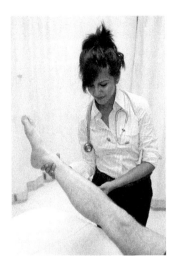

Figure 12.5 Buerger's test.

 NB Reactive hyperaemia is a transient increase in blood flow that develops following a period of ischaemia. It is caused by accumulation of vasodilatory metabolites (such as nitrous oxide) during the period of hypoxia. The leg will develop a red colour, and this is a sign of peripheral arterial disease.

To complete the examination

- Offer to perform a full cardiac examination
- Perform a full neurological examination of the lower limbs
- Check ankle brachial pressure index
- Thank the patient
- Ensure the patient is covered up and comfortable

OSCE Key Learning Points

Ankle brachial pressure index (ABPI)

✔ *Normal*: >1

✔ *Claudication*: 0.4–0.7

✔ *Critical ischaemia*: 0.1–0.4

✔ Arterial calcification (e.g. in diabetes mellitus) can cause an artificial increase in ABPI

OSCE Key Learning Points

Peripheral arterial system: example presentation

✔ I was asked to examine Mr Jones, a 67-year-old man who presented with leg pain.

✔ On general examination he was alert and orientated and comfortable at rest. On inspection of the peripheries, there was obvious tar staining and corneal arcus. Pulse was 80 bpm and regular, and there was no palpable abdominal aortic aneurysm.

✔ Examining the lower limbs, on inspection they were pale in colour bilaterally, with a thin and shiny appearance of the skin and hair loss. There was an ulcer on the lateral border of the left foot which was 2 cm in diameter and had a regular border with a punched out appearance. On palpation, the feet were cold and capillary refill time was increased, at 4 seconds on the left and 3 seconds on the right. Femoral and popliteal pulses were present bilaterally. On the right side, posterior tibial and dorsalis pulses were weak but palpable. On the left side, both posterior tibial and dorsalis pulses were impalpable. Doppler auscultation confirmed presence of the left posterior tibial pulse, which was monophasic, but the left dorsalis pedis pulse was absent to Doppler auscultation.

✔ I would like to complete my examination by performing a neurological examination of the lower limbs, and by measuring the ankle brachial pressure index.

✔ In summary, this gentleman demonstrates signs consistent with peripheral arterial disease. The presence of tissue loss in the form of an ulcer indicates stage 4 disease according to the Fontaine classification.

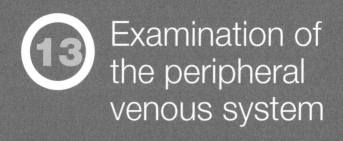

Examination of the peripheral venous system

13

OSCE Key Learning Points

✔ Remember to spend time inspecting from the end of the bed

Preparation

- *Cross infection*: wash and dry hands, bare below the elbow
- *Introductions*: yourself and the task; confirm patient's name and age
- *Consent*: to the procedure
- *Pain*: is the patient in pain
- *Privacy*: ensure privacy, e.g. curtains drawn around bed
- *Position*: ideally standing initially
- *Exposure*: from the waist down, underwear on

End of bed inspection

- *Environment*: glyceryl trinitrate (GTN) spray, oxygen, walking aids
- *Patient*: breathlessness, distress

Medical Student Survival Skills: Clinical Examination, First Edition. Philip Jevon, Elliot Epstein,
Sarah Mensforth, and Caroline MacMahon.
© 2020 John Wiley & Sons Ltd. Published 2020 by John Wiley & Sons Ltd.
Companion website: www.wiley.com/go/jevon/medicalstudent

The peripheries

See Chapter 12

The lower limbs

Inspection

- Colour
- Oedema: press over medial malleolus, then move proximally to determine how far up the leg it reaches
- Inverted champagne bottle appearance (due to lipodermatosclerosis of the gaiter area)
- Atrophie blanche
- Spider veins
- Venous eczema
- Discoloration: due to deposition of haemosiderin, a red blood cell break-down product, which is extravasated into the dermis through damaged capillaries
- Varicosities: note distribution and likely veins involved
- Ulcers: commonly in the gaiter area
- Saphenofemoral junction (SFJ): look for saphena varix

 NB Knowledge of the lower limb venous system is helpful (Figure 13.1).

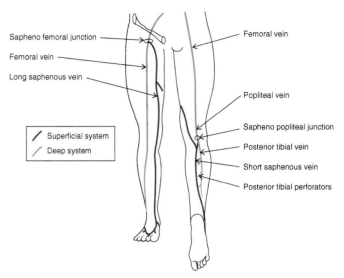

Figure 13.1 Venous anatomy.

Palpation

- Temperature
- Oedema
  - Ask about ankle pain
  - Gently press thumb over the medial malleolus for 2 seconds
  - If indentation is observed, move proximally to establish the level of oedema
- Palpate varicosities for tenderness: may indicate thrombophlebitis
- Palpate along course of long and short saphenous veins
  - There may be varicosities that are not obvious on inspection but which can be palpated
- Lipodermatosclerosis: may be visible but more evident on palpation. Most commonly found in the gaiter area
- Pulses (dorsalis pedis and posterior tibial): a quick screening test for arterial disease, which often coexists
- SFJ for saphenous varix

OSCE Key Learning Points

✔ The SFJ is located 3–4 cm inferolateral to the pubic tubercle. It is essential to locate and examine this landmark in your assessment

OSCE Key Learning Points

Risk factors for varicose veins include

✔ Obesity

✔ Family history

✔ Pregnancy

✔ Pelvic mass

✔ Previous deep vein thrombosis (DVT)

Handheld Doppler ultrasound

The aim of this investigation is to identify the location of venous incompetence.

• Hold the Doppler at the SPJ, located in the popliteal fossa, lateral to the popliteal pulse

- Squeeze the calf
- One 'whoosh' should be heard as the venous blood returns proximally (Figure 13.2a). This is normal
- When you release the calf, a competent vein should prevent venous backflow, therefore there should be no further sound
- Retrograde flow is audible if there is venous incompetence, i.e. there is a second 'whoosh' (Figure 13.2b)
- A positive test here suggests disease of the short saphenous vein

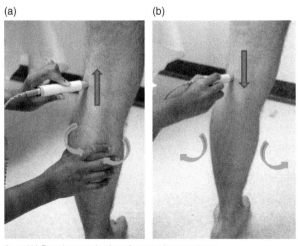

Figure 13.2 (a and b) Doppler examination of venous incompetence.

- Hold the Doppler at the SFJ, located 4 cm inferior to the femoral pulsation
  - Squeeze the calf
  - A positive test here indicates disease of the SFJ or long saphenous vein

NB Limitations of Doppler ultrasound: while this examination is more sensitive than the historical clinical tests, it does not allow visualisation of the vein in question, therefore it is not possible to say with complete confidence from where the flow is originating.

Special tests

These tests have been superseded by handheld Doppler ultrasound, and hence are no longer routinely performed in clinical practice. If you choose to perform them, you should make it clear to the examiner that you understand this.

- *Trendelenburg's test*: start with the patient supine, and confirm that they have no pain in their hip. Raise the leg in question to 45° to empty the veins. Apply pressure to the area of the SFJ (with your hand or a tourniquet), then ask the patient to stand. Watch carefully to see if their varicosities refill on standing. If they quickly refill, you have not controlled the incompetent veins, therefore they are assumed to be distal to the SFJ. If the varicosities fail to refill quickly on standing, incompetence at the SFJ is suggested. The tourniquet test uses the same routine, with the tourniquet moved more distally with each repetition, to determine the level at which incompetent valves are found
- *Tap test*: perform this with the patient standing. Palpate the SFJ, while tapping the long saphenous vein at the level medial to the knee. Palpation of transmitted impulses to the SFJ indicate incompetence of veins along the long saphenous vein

OSCE Key Learning Points

Complications of chronic venous insufficiency include
- ✔ Pain
- ✔ Ulceration
- ✔ Thrombophlebitis
- ✔ Cellulitis
- ✔ DVT

To complete the examination

- Cardiovascular examination, particularly if the patient has peripheral oedema
- Full arterial examination of the lower limb
- Abdominal examination and digital rectal examination (DRE) (for masses)
- Ankle brachial pressure index (ABPI) (see Chapter 12)
- Duplex ultrasound examination of the superficial and deep veins
- Thank the patient
- Cover the patient up and ensure they are comfortable

NB ABPI is essential to rule out concurrent arterial insufficiency, as this is a contraindication to compression therapy.

OSCE Key Learning Points

Peripheral venous system: example presentation

✔ I was asked to examine Mrs Jones, an 83-year-old lady who presents with pain and swelling in the lower limbs, worsened by standing.

✔ On end of bed inspection, she was alert and well and comfortable at rest, and a walking stick was noted by the bed.

✔ On inspection of the lower limbs, there was mild swelling, with brown discoloration of the medial ankle and anterior lower leg bilaterally. There were dilated and tortuous vessels noted on the left lateral lower leg, from the popliteal fossa to the posterior lateral malleolus, which would fit the distribution of the short saphenous vein. There were no ulcers.

✔ On palpation, temperature was normal, and there was bilateral pitting oedema to the mid calf. Varicosities were soft and non-tender, and there was no palpable lipodermatosclerosis. Pulses were present.

✔ Handheld Doppler examination was normal at the saphenofemoral junction, but there was audible incompetence at the level of the saphenopopliteal junction on the left hand side.

✔ In summary, this lady shows signs of chronic venous insufficiency, with incompetence apparent in the left short saphenous vein. I would like to further investigate this by requesting a departmental duplex ultrasound evaluation of the lower limb venous system, to adequately evaluate the deep, superficial, and perforator veins.

OSCE Key Learning Points

Clinical signs of deep vein thrombosis
- ✔ Tenderness
- ✔ Erythema
- ✔ Swelling
- ✔ Increased temperature
- ✔ The patient with a DVT may not display all these signs, and the clinical presentation can be subtle. Take a thorough history enquiring about risk factors, and maintain a low threshold of suspicion

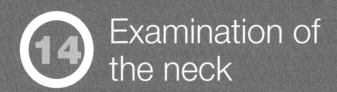

14 Examination of the neck

OSCE Key Learning Points

✔ Remember to spend time inspecting from the end of the bed

NB Remember to follow the examiner's command:
- 'Examine the patient's neck' – start with the neck
- 'Examine the patient's thyroid status' – you need to include the peripheries

Preparation

- *Cross infection*: wash and dry hands, bare below the elbow
- *Introductions*: yourself and the task; confirm patient's name and age
- *Consent*: to the procedure
- *Pain*: is the patient in pain
- *Privacy*: ensure privacy, e.g. curtains drawn around bed
- *Position*: ideally sitting out in a chair – access behind the chair will be required
- *Exposure*: the head and neck should be fully exposed, no collars, high neck clothing, jewellery, etc.

Medical Student Survival Skills: Clinical Examination, First Edition. Philip Jevon, Elliot Epstein, Sarah Mensforth, and Caroline MacMahon.
© 2020 John Wiley & Sons Ltd. Published 2020 by John Wiley & Sons Ltd.
Companion website: www.wiley.com/go/jevon/medicalstudent

End of bed inspection

- *Environment*: fluid restriction, glyceryl trinitrate (GTN) spray, oxygen, infusions, cardiac monitor
- *Patient*: breathlessness, distress, position, orthopnoea, pallor

The peripheries

- *Patient*: hoarse voice, respiratory distress, anxious state, tremor, body mass index (BMI)

The neck

Inspection
- Inspect from the front and sides
- Inspect for the six 'S's:
  - Site, size, shape, symmetry, skin, scars
- If there is a midline mass, proceed to do two tests:
  - Watch for movement with swallowing a sip of water– a thyroid mass
  - Watch for upward movement on tongue protrusion – a thyroglossal mass

NB If there is an *obvious mass* on inspection, proceed to examine this mass as in the next section. If there is *no obvious mass*, proceed to the routine lymph node examination given later in this chapter.

Palpation
- Standing behind the patient, examine the normal side first. Then compare the abnormal side

OSCE Key Learning Points

How to palpate the neck

✔ Figure 14.1 shows how to palpate: standing behind the patient, using the flats of your fingertips, make small circular motions to appreciate the densities of the subcutaneous tissues beneath.

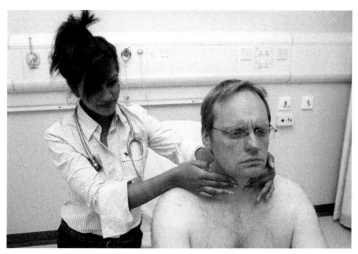

Figure 14.1 Neck examination.

- Examine the features of the mass:
  - Surface
  - Edge
  - Consistency
  - Mobility (fixing to the skin)
  - Fluctuance
  - Pulsatility
  - Reducibility
  - Transilluminability
- If the mass is midline, you can repeat the tests of swallowing water and tongue protrusion whilst palpating.
- Assess for movement of a thyroglossal mass on tongue protrusion (Figure 14.2)

Percussion
- If the inferior border of the mass cannot be felt, the mass may extend into the chest
- Percuss the mass comparing the percussion note to the resonant lung

Auscultation
- A large thyroid mass may have an extensive blood supply, resulting in a bruit
- Auscultate over the central mass

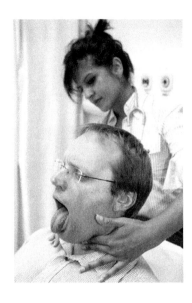

Figure 14.2 Assessing for movement of a thyroglossal mass on tongue protrusion.

Examination of the lymph nodes

If there is no obvious mass on inspection proceed to routine palpation of all lymph nodes. The scheme suggested below will help missing any groups (Figure 14.3). If a mass is found during this, examine this using the scheme given earlier.

- Start at the sternoclavicular joint. Palpate the anterior border of the sterno-cleidomastoid muscle (**a** in Figure 14.3b – pre-tracheal and anterior cervical lymph nodes) and continue superiorly
- Once at the ear lobe, proceed along the inner inferior border of the mandible towards the mental protuberances (**b** – submandibular; **c** – submental lymph nodes)
- From there, move posteriorly to examine the pre-auricular area (**d** – pre-auricular lymph nodes)
- Palpate the posterior auricular area (**e** – post-auricular lymph nodes)
- Palpate inferiorly down the posterior border of the sternocleidomastoid muscle (**f** – posterior cervical lymph nodes) to the clavicle
- Palpate laterally along the superior border of the clavicle (**g** –supraclavicular lymph nodes) to the trapezius muscle
- Palpate superiorly along the lateral border of the trapezius (posterior cervical) towards the base of the skull (**h** – occipital lymph nodes)

(a)   (b)

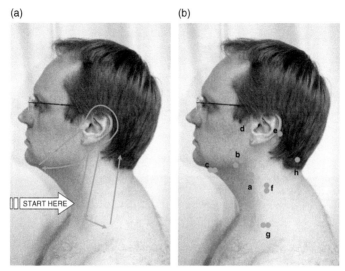

Figure 14.3 (a and b) Location of the cervical lymph nodes and a systematic approach to examination (**a–h**).

If there is a thyroid mass …?

- After completing the examination of the neck, if there is a thyroid mass, complete an assessment of thyroid status. Begin at the hands and proceed through the examination of peripheries – general appearance, hands, and face (Table 14.1).

Table 14.1 Features of Hyperthyroidism and Hypothyroidism

	Features of hyperthyroidism	Features of hypothyroidism
General appearance	Anxious, restless, low BMI	Tired, sleepy, high BMI, thinning hair
Hands	Tremor, warm, sweaty, tachycardic pulse or atrial fibrillation	Cool, bradycardic pulse
Face		Greasy skin – peaches and cream
Eyes	Graves' disease only: lid lag, lid retraction, proptosis, exophthalmos	Enophthalmos
Others	Graves' disease only: pretibial myxoedema, proximal myopathy	Slow relaxing reflexes, proximal myopathy

To complete the examination

If there is a thyroid mass
- Offer to examine or question to ascertain thyroid status

If there is another neck mass
- Examine the ear, nose, and throat
- Examine the other groups of lymph nodes – axillary, groin
- Thank the patient
- Ensure the patient is covered up and comfortable

OSCE Key Learning Points

The neck: example presentation

✔ I examined this elderly lady's neck. There was nothing to note on inspection, with no scars or skin changes. On examination there is a single, well-defined, 2 cm, hard lump in the right anterior triangle of the neck in the submandibular area, adjacent to the angle of the mandible. This was not tethered to the skin, and was non-tender. There were no other masses.

✔ To complete the examination I would examine the ear, nose, and throat and the other lymph node groups.

15 Examination of the breast

Preparation

- *Cross infection*: wash and dry hands, bare below the elbow
- *Introductions*: yourself and the task; confirm patient's name and age
- *Consent*: to the procedure
- *Pain*: is the patient in pain?
- *Privacy*: ensure privacy, e.g. curtains drawn around bed; chaperone
- *Position*: initially sitting on the edge of the bed
- *Exposure*: from the waist up

 NB Make sure there is a chaperone in attendence.

Medical Student Survival Skills: Clinical Examination, First Edition. Philip Jevon, Elliot Epstein, Sarah Mensforth, and Caroline MacMahon.
© 2020 John Wiley & Sons Ltd. Published 2020 by John Wiley & Sons Ltd.
Companion website: www.wiley.com/go/jevon/medicalstudent

End of bed inspection

- *Environment*: medications, oxygen
- *Patient*: pain, distress, position, general health

 NB When informed about an abnormality, examine the normal breast first.

  ✔ During examination, observe the patient's face for pain

Inspection

Ask the patient to sit on the edge of the bed, with her hands on her hips.

Inspection of the breasts:
- Asymmetry
- Lumps or swellings
- Nipple abnormalities, e.g. inversion
- Skin changes, e.g. peau d'orange, eczema
- Discharge from nipple
- Prominent veins
- Signs of previous breast cancer, e.g. mastectomy, scars, and hair loss

Also inspect:
- Supraclavicular regions and axillae for lymphadenopathy, veins, and muscle wasting
- Arms for lymphoedema

Repeat the above inspection with each of the following two positions:
- Arms down and relaxed
- Hands behind the head, elbows pushed back

Palpation

 NB Ensure you ask the patient if she experiences any pain during examination.

Breasts

- Ask the patient to lie on the couch at 45° and position her hand behind her head on the side of the breast you are examining first (the normal one)
- Examine the four breast quadrants: place your (warmed up) hand flat on the breast, beginning from outside and working towards the nipple. Remember that breast tissue extends towards the axilla
- Palpate the nipples and check for discharge

Axilla

- Ask the patient to place her forearm on top of your forearm
- Palpate for lymphadenopathy in the four walls of the axilla (anterior, posterior, medial, lateral) and in the apex

Supraclavicular fossa

- Palpate for lymphadenopathy in the supraclavicular fossa

Repeat the above palpation procedures for the other breast. If a lump is found, describe it in relation to tenderness, site, size, shape, temperature, reducibility, mobility, and tethering.

OSCE Key Learning Points

Biopsies for breast lumps
- ✔ Fine needle aspiration cytology
- ✔ Core (Tru-Cut) biopsy
- ✔ Surgical biopsy

To complete the examination

- If a lump is found, offer to examine other systems, e.g. respiratory system
- Thank the patient
- Make sure the patient is covered up and comfortable

OSCE Key Learning Points

Warning signs of breast cancer
- ✔ An area that is distinctly different from any other area on either breast
- ✔ A lump, bumpy area or thickening in or near the breast or in the underarm area that persists through the menstrual cycle

✔ A change in breast size, shape, or contour, particularly those caused by arm movements or by lifting the breasts

✔ A mass or lump, which may feel as small as a pea

✔ A difference in the feel or appearance of the breast or nipple (skin becomes dimpled, puckered, scaly, red, or inflamed)

✔ Discomfort or pain in one breast that is new and persists

✔ Blood-stained or clear fluid discharge from a nipple

✔ Any change in nipple position – e.g. inverted or pointing differently

OSCE Key Learning Points

Location of breast tumours

✔ 41% upper outer quadrant

✔ 14% upper inner quadrant

✔ 5% lower inner quadrant

✔ 6% lower outer quadrant

✔ 34% in the area behind the nipple

OSCE Key Learning Points

The breast: example presentation

✔ This is Mrs Smith, a 50-year-old lady who presents with a lump in her left breast.

✔ On general examination she is alert and orientated and comfortable at rest, with no obvious peripheral stigmata of disease.

✔ On inspection of the breasts, there are no visible scars, erythema, or any other abnormalities. However, on palpation I palpated a pea-type structure in the upper outer quadrant of the left breast.

✔ To complete my examination, I would examine the lymph nodes in the axilla and neck and I would order appropriate investigations, e.g. chest X-ray.

Index

Note: Page numbers in *italics* refer to figures.
Page numbers in **bold** refer to tables.

Medical Student Survival Skills: Clinical Examination, First Edition. Philip Jevon, Elliot Epstein,
Sarah Mensforth, and Caroline MacMahon.
© 2020 John Wiley & Sons Ltd. Published 2020 by John Wiley & Sons Ltd.
Companion website: www.wiley.com/go/jevon/medicalstudent